HARD TO SWALLOW

Charleston, SC
www.PalmettoPublishing.com

Hard To Swallow
Copyright © 2021 by Hamlin Emory, MD

First Edition

Paperback ISBN: 978-1-64990-840-7
Hardcover ISBN: 978-1-64990-841-4
eBook ISBN: 978-1-64990-842-1

HARD TO SWALLOW

FROM SUPERSTITION TO PSYCHIATRY

HAMLIN EMORY, MD
As told to and edited by A. J. Adelman

FOREWORD

I met Dr. Hamlin Emory in the early 1990's. He was the medical director and a psychiatrist at a hospital where I was hired to develop and serve as clinical director for an eating disorder unit. What stood out immediately was his dapper style and scholarly grasp of language. Over time, I observed his deep commitment and rigor in finding and improving any neurophysiology that was involved in each patient's suffering. Through my relationship with Dr. Emory, I came to understand a new way of looking at my clinical practice as a therapist and helping my patients recover.

Dr. Emory introduced me to a new paradigm, one that measures different brainwave frequencies as a way to help diagnose and treat mental disorders. As he once told me, "Carolyn, my job is to give the patient a full deck of cards to play with. Yours is to help them learn how to play the cards to their best advantage." Over the last 30 years his statement has been true and his method has been astonishingly successful.

The first time I sent Dr. Emory a patient, it was an eye-opening event. He was a 20-year-old male patient,

"Ron," who suffered with bulimia nervosa and also had a variety of other diagnoses and complications. In addition to his eating disorder, he had been diagnosed as bipolar. Yet, the medication was not helping. Also, he was ashamed to admit that he had a problem with bed wetting. I decided to send him to Dr. Emory.

After consulting with Ron, and performing an EEG/QEEG, Dr. Emory prescribed a very different medical regimen. Ron stopped bed wetting immediately and his mood swings and manic episodes, which had been the most destructive in his life, ceased. With these things abated, he was then able to focus on his eating disorder behaviors and begin the process of recovery.

I was astounded.

This began a long collaboration with Dr. Emory that included hiring him as the consulting psychiatrist for the first ever residential treatment center for eating disorders, Monte Nido, opened in 1996. Without a doubt, Dr. Emory's contribution to patient care at my facility was critical in achieving the outstanding outcomes and extremely high recovery rates.

During the next two decades together, I learned over and over again, that underlying brain abnormalities in a patient's EEG/QEEG contributed to their maladaptive behaviors in ways that were crucial in understanding and helping them recover. Looking at a patient's EEG/QEEG we could see patterns, such as the need for a "stimulant" medication that was considered antithetical by standard psychiatric practice; yet for such individuals, it was calming, stopped their automatic foot tapping behaviors, and actually helped with, rather than interfered with, their appetite.

I learned that Prozac, routinely prescribed for patients with eating disorders, was contraindicated in many individuals according to their brain EEG/QEEG data and in fact, after a short period of a positive response, actually made these patients worse. In addition, I worked with Dr. Emory to find natural supplements that would help normalize EEG/QEEG patterns similar to those that medications could correct. I observed some people who were able to discontinue their medication and substitute a regimen of "over the counter" supplements.

Finally, I am a testament to the benefits of Dr. Emory's method. I decided early on to go through the process of having Dr. Emory give me an EEG/QEEG and analyze it. When he called me afterwards, he held up the results and said, "Carolyn, let this be a testament to your character."

It turned out my EEG/QEEG pattern showed two variants that indicated I was a candidate for an activating medication. I remember thinking, "I like myself, I feel fine, why would I want to change myself?" But Dr. Emory asked me to simply try the medication and see how I felt. So, I did.

I took the medicine and did not tell anyone. I did not notice anything, but two days later my husband said, "What is going on with you? Normally you buzz around here on high speed and yet now you seem much calmer and balanced." I was shocked.

I told him about the new medication, and he replied, "Well, I think it is good for you." I had not really noticed and I was not sure he was right...so I stopped taking the medication and again did not tell anyone. Sure enough, no more than two days went by when my husband asked, "Have you stopped taking the medication?"

Wow! So I restarted the medication and it became clear that with Dr. Emory's prescription, I was better able to focus, was calmer and apparently easier to live with.

Dr. Emory's method is not a panacea for all patients. I still think that therapists are important and I believe my work is valid and valuable. However, I also know now that in the field of mental health, we are lagging behind. Because people do not understand the usefulness of EEG/QEEG, we are failing with many patients who could benefit from EEG/QEEG technology and Dr. Emory's therapeutic method.

I often tell Dr. Emory that, like Van Gogh, he is ahead of his time; and it is likely that he will not see the value of his work fully appreciated in his lifetime. Meanwhile, I am one of many professionals who have seen the importance of his work and will continue to recommend his method to patients as needed.

Carolyn Costin
The Carolyn Costin Institute
Author, *8 Keys to Recovery from an Eating Disorder*,
***The Eating Disorder Sourcebook* and more.**

DEDICATION

*To my wife, Virginia, whose inspiration and tireless devotion
to my work made this book a reality.*

BRAIN 1 STTM

"A healthy brain automatically balances itself and the body 24/7; yet, inherited differences in brain function can impair these interactions and cause persistent distress. Brain 1st™ uses measurable, biological parameters and thus is a fact-driven way to improve brain function that has caused physical illness, learning problems, substance dependence or a mental disorder. Each person's treatment is personalized and selected to achieve brain-body balance."

Hamlin Emory, MD

The Emory Method is based on the research of E. Roy John, Ph.D. and his associates, who spent nearly a decade acquiring (visual) EEG and (quantitative) QEEG data in healthy children and adults between the ages of 6 and 80. Dr. John's database was FDA approved in 1994. Just as cardiologists use the EKG (electrocardiogram) to measure heart function, the EEG/QEEG technology provide a lab test to understand each patient's Brain Electrical Activity. Dr. Emory has been using this data since the 1980s to restore patients to optimal wellbeing.

TABLE OF CONTENTS

PROLOGUE

During my early years as a psychiatrist, I witnessed the physical and mental suffering of others and lamented the intensity of their agony. I grieved for the parents who lost their children. I anguished over the thousands who suffered from mood disorders, migraines, drug addiction and a host of other ailments that render them unable to work or live a healthy life. I gradually realized that all the years of medical training had not prepared me to understand the underlying physical aspects of mental illnesses.

Over time, I became convinced that the psychiatric community separated people into personality types without sufficient physical data. Doctors assumed that their patient's symptoms and behaviors were the result of warped personalities. It took me about a decade to realize that a person's repetitive and dysfunctional behaviors were their therapeutic attempts to reduce his or her misery. Those who repeatedly fail their doctor's treatment are labeled "treatment resistant." My belief is that these patients are improperly diagnosed. Invisible illnesses confront doctors every day, and often patients and doctors alike feel helpless in the face of unyielding failure; however, blaming victims for their invisible illness is cruel.

Traditional psychiatric practice veered away from the medical model decades ago, a model all physicians learn in their medical training. Healthy people enjoy predictable physical and mental wellbeing, yet, those with chronic mental disorders and substance abuse do not have such capacity. This is why people with brain-based mental disorders find other ways to relieve their agony. Some choose alcohol. Others resort to street drugs. But all look for a self-medicating way to feel better. While these self-treatments work for a short period of time, they do not address the underlying cause of a patient's dysfunction.

Traditional psychiatrists do not examine people. They prefer focusing on what the patients tell them instead of measuring the brain function they are treating. They stigmatize their patients' behavior, giving them a diagnosis without any corresponding physical data. These diagnoses are names describing the person's symptoms and behaviors and are recorded on their medical record, following patients throughout their lives. If doctors would gather physical evidence to see if the patient has an inherited variance in the automatic circuits of his or her brain, they might discover an otherwise invisible dysfunction, irregularity or abnormality causing the patient's suffering. Since psychiatrists do not physically examine their patients thoroughly, they usually have little data to support their diagnosis or treatment plan. Sometimes doctors get lucky with their educated guessing. Often, they just make their patients "less worse."

This is my story about how a comprehensive medical approach and EEG/QEEG measures helped me transition from the psychiatric model (treating symptoms and behaviors), to the medical model, which includes functional brain measures, and through experience improved patient's physical health and mental wellbeing.

CHAPTER 1

A HARD PILL TO SWALLOW

In 1970, I was working in Sigonella Naval Hospital in Italy. I can replay the scene in my mind as if it took place yesterday. The week before, a mother had brought her seven-year-old son in due to hyperactivity and lack of sleep. At the time, he had no physical abnormalities, so I prescribed a common antidepressant to alleviate his symptoms.

A week later, the mother returned very upset. During the appointment, she admonished me for the medication I had prescribed.

"Dr. Emory, at first, he took the pill," the mother told me. "But after a week, he now spits it out every time."

She then demonstrated what she had just described, plopping him on the exam table, thrusting the tablet into his mouth and clamping his head and jaw together like a vice to keep his mouth shut.

I watched in astonishment as he writhed in protest with dilated pupils and a reddening face; still, the tablet emerged between his pursed lips and fell onto the floor.

"See doctor! 'Brian' won't swallow it!"

She was desperate. I had never seen a child, or an adult, steadfastly refuse a medication. For a moment, I was speechless. Then, I recalled Aristotle's opinion that "people seek what is desirable and avoid what is undesirable."

I believed the boy had swallowed the pill for almost a week; then, as the medication's concentration reached a maximum threshold in his brain, the child experienced a negative sensation and promptly expelled it.

It was apparent to me that the medication I prescribed didn't fit his physiology!

Attempting to reassure her, I said, "Your child's refusal is his way of telling us the medication doesn't agree with him. Unfortunately, when we prescribe medications for conditions of the brain, there are no lab tests to prove whether it is helping or not. It's trial and error."

At the time, I knew nothing about the budding field of electroencephalography (EEG), which tracks and records brain wave patterns and is used to find problems associated with the brain's electrical activity. The use of EEGs was not emphasized in my psychiatric courses. In fact, I never observed a psychiatrist physically examine a patient during my four years of psychiatric training. My professors were devotees of Freud, Jung and a long list of other prominent theorists. Their treatment was not based on differences in brain activity. Their approach was like being a stranger in a strange land. They had separated the brain from the body and focused on treating symptoms and behaviors. As a result, the effects of prescribed medications on the brain were forgotten.

While I was trained to observe illnesses such as depression, anorexia, anxiety and bipolar disorder, none of these labels are medical diagnoses. They are constructs. This disconnect held clues to brain function and behavior. The omission was now obvious to me and came from being trained as a general practitioner before becoming a psychiatrist. My goal to bridge the disconnect resulted in a lifelong journey to find the physiology in mental and behavioral disorders.

CHAPTER 2

FROM SUPERSTITION TO PSYCHIATRY

Before the European Enlightenment of the 18th century, religious doctrines generally defined what was good and bad conduct.

Consider these 17th-century English behavioral categories:

- **Normal individuals:** Those who only occasionally and momentarily lose their reason
- **Natural fools:** Those irresponsible since birth
- **The insane:** Those who were at one time normal, but now crazy
- **Lunatics:** Insane people who occasionally recover their reason

Now, consider these 18th-century French behavioral categories:

- **Raving lunatics:** (or maniacs)
- **Quiet lunatics:** (to be confined, not tied up)
- **Eccentrics:** (to be watched over constantly)
- **The insane:** (with unpredictable behavior)
- **Imbeciles:** (to be directed like children)

- **Demented lunatics:** (to be cared for physically)
- **Normal individuals:** not described

Citation: Beyond the Unconscious; Essays of Henri F. Ellenberger in the History of Psychiatry; Pages 312 - 313; Copyright 1993; Published by Princeton University Press, 41 William Street, Princeton, New Jersey 08540

Imagine living in the mid-1700s. A fever was thought to be the result of exorcizing a demon in the body!

The discovery by the son of a Lutheran minister and professor at the University of Berlin would make a ground-breaking discovery. Johann Christian Reil was the first medical doctor to teach that abnormalities of the nervous system could disrupt awareness and cause abnormal perceptions, thoughts and behaviors.

Early in his career, Reil lived with an older professor, whose early onset of dementia caused him to awaken each morning in a delusional state. He began each day walking about his spacious mansion looking for a crazy person; however, by late afternoon, he realized that the crazy person he sought was really himself.

Reil's first book appeared in 1802. *Fieberhafte Nervenkrankheiten* (Feverish Nervous Illness) was about feverish patients whose subsequent thinking, behavior and personality became radically altered. Without knowledge of individual brain function, Reil declared that some mental illnesses are "…caused by forces in the nervous system which are totally unknown," but rendered a person incapable of accurately comprehending reality. This observation was a revolutionary one!

Around this time, and in the early decades of the newly minted United States of America, Dr. Benjamin Rush

(1746–1813), professor of medicine at the University of Pennsylvania, also inferred that physiologic causes existed for some psychiatric illnesses.

Dr. Rush was a Renaissance man. Narcissistic, yet socially liberal, his zeal for controversial medical treatments occasionally eclipsed his judgment. For instance, Dr. Rush was an ardent advocate of bloodletting, the medical benefit of which was debatable at the time and later deemed largely harmful.

After retiring as the first president of the United States, George Washington became afflicted with a severe throat infection requiring medical care. Dr. Rush arranged a treatment plan that included bleeding the illness out of the President. Tragically, the procedure caused dehydration and impaired his immune system, and as a result, President Washington subsequently died. While bloodletting would prove to be a point of controversy on his otherwise illustrious career, his contribution to modern psychiatry is indisputable.

In a letter to President John Adams, Dr. Rush penned, "I am convinced that these disorders will be found subject to the same physical laws as other medical illnesses..." In the next chapter, I will provide an example of my own journey to understanding the brain-body connection.

CHAPTER 3

BORN A LEFTY

I was born with three congenital defects: The first is a difference in length between my right and left legs; the second is torticollis, a fibrotic segment of the sterno-cleido-mastoid (SCM) muscle on the right side of my neck, and the third is a mild scoliosis of my lower back. The leg difference was only apparent to a tailor who measured me for new trousers, but the fibrotic muscle caused my head to tilt about 15 degrees beyond the normal vertical position.

Throughout my early school years, my peers relentlessly teased me, assuming I was adopting a cocky pose. I was considered an odd ball, which concerned my parents. When I was in the fourth grade, my doctor ordered weekly physical therapy to stretch the muscle in my neck that was causing the tilt, but a year later, there was no change. While some physiological aspects are worth changing, others are not. And my parents knew how to distinguish between the two.

I was born left-handed. Being a lefty did not pose a problem for me until I entered grade school, whereupon my first-grade teacher struck my left hand each time I tried to write with it. Several days passed before I told Mother about this practice. She was visibly shaken.

The following morning, and without a word, mother took me by the hand and walked me to school. She marched stridently into the principal's office as I sheepishly followed behind her. After requesting a word with the principal, we were ushered into his office.

"What can I do for you today, Mrs. Emory?" he asked with a smile.

"Good Morning, Mr. Saunders. My son, Warden Hamlin, tells me that he is being struck on his left hand every day in school. Are you aware of this practice?"

Mr. Saunders replied, "While I wasn't privy to the specific event you're describing, I'm not surprised, Mrs. Emory. We encourage our children to use their right hand."

Mother responded forcefully as she leaned forward with a respectful smile, "The Good Lord made my son left-handed, and left-handed my son shall remain. Do we understand each other, Mr. Saunders?"

Taken aback, he replied, "Yes, Mrs. Emory, we certainly do."

That incident depicts how my parents handled most matters—with quiet dignity and respect. I still aspire every day to emulate their example.

One summer morning, Mother drove me in the family Studebaker to the Medical College of Virginia in downtown Richmond. After a physical exam and x-rays, the orthopedic surgeon said, "The only way to correct your son's tilted head is to surgically remove the fibrosis that is causing it." The ensuing discussion between the surgeon and my mother was overshadowed by a growing sense of dread. My mind assaulted me with fantasies of mutilation and bleeding to death.

After much discussion, my parents detailed their plan of action. "On Wednesday, you will be admitted to the hospital. Thursday morning, an anesthesiologist will give you medication so you can sleep. You will not feel any pain during the operation. When it is over, you will wake up in your room. A money tree will be placed on your eating tray. Visitors will pin a few dollars on it during their visits. Your head will soon become vertical, and within a week, you will return home." And so, it was.

Fear vanished! It was remarkable. I became curious about the procedure, hospital, operating room, anesthesia, doctors and nurses. Despite pre-operative medication, I remember asking many questions as I was rolled into the operating room and lifted onto the table. Suddenly I was unconscious.

I awakened that afternoon with no memory of the operation. I had a substantial bandage over the right side of my neck, and a roommate, Mr. Wolff, was in the adjoining bed. My mother told me that Mr. Wolff had been a citizen of Austria and during WWII, forced to stay in one of Adolf Hitler's concentration camps. In the ensuing months, Mr. Wolff never talked about the death camps, yet our conversations have endured.

Mr. Wolff was a wise, cultured and gentle man. In hindsight, he was a grandfatherly figure during that week in the hospital. In subsequent months, Mother and I visited him and his wife in their downtown Richmond apartment. I did not know that he was dying of colon cancer. Six months later, it took his life, but not my memory of him.

Being a successful patient at the age of 10 catalyzed my confidence and inspired interest in becoming a medical doctor, particularly a surgeon. Now, my head's position, whether I was sitting or standing, was vertical like everyone else's and my peers' bullying about being "cocky" ceased. But I noted something new and unexpected with my new, vertical head pose. My view of the external world now tilted to the left. When I tilted my head to the right as it had been, the external world was horizontal again. I concluded that my brain was playing tricks on me.

The surgeon had not prepared me for this phenomenon, but I wasn't afraid and didn't speak of it to anyone. For weeks, I purposely oscillated between the two head positions when I was alone, trying my new, vertical head mode and regressing to the former tilted mode. Gradually, I concluded that since my vision had seemed "straight" with a tilted head, my vision would likely become horizontal again over time. I said nothing about this to anyone, waiting to see what would happen. I had an "optimistic belief about the potential of physiologic change." As I suspected, some months later my visual field straightened.

Today I understand this phenomenon as the neuroplasticity of the brain, which gradually corrected itself as my head position changed. After recovering from the operation, I returned to school and wrote an essay about becoming a medical doctor. Eventually, exploring the brain-body connection would become my professional passion. But this perspective stood in stark opposition to the widely accepted position initially championed by Sigmund Freud.

Born in 1856, Sigmund Freud was a trained neurologist, who abandoned the medical model and popularized a "talking treatment" called psychoanalysis.

While clocks, watches, stethoscopes and blood pressure monitors were available at the time to treat patients, he did not use them. Rather than rely on physical examinations, Freud assumed that people's neurotic conflicts, drives and instincts were the cause of their maladaptive behavior and symptoms. He ignored the notion that his patients might have been physically ill. Although he used the terms "instinct" and "drive," Freud ignored the physiology in mentality. He asserted that psychoanalysis could relieve the suffering of abnormal instincts without a physical examination.

Although Freud was a physician, his focus was not on physiology but on emotional states. Freud's position was that everyone's brain was fundamentally the same, and what distinguished one brain from another is a person's experiences and memories. While one's conditioning plays a significant role, it does not provide information about individual brain function.

Overall, Freud's theories were infused with his opinions and conjectures that lacked rigorous scientific inquiry. His observations often reflected a negative bias and assumed the worst in people. Viewed from a contemporary perspective, Freud's theories reveal his limited understanding of human physiology. Freud is the father of the *brain-body disconnect.* While his theories would shake up psychiatry forever, his major blind spot of ignoring brain states would call into question many of his findings. In the next chapter, we will learn how important brain states are.

CHAPTER 4

EXTROVERTS, INTROVERTS, NEUROTICS AND PSYCHOTICS

Hans Eysenck, PhD, was the most published neuropsychologist in the 20th century. A giant in this field, he understood that differences in brain activity influence differences in personality. Eysenck delineated the four temperaments, coining the following terms:

- Extrovert
- Introvert
- Neurotic
- Psychotic

In addition, he recognized that visual EEG patterns provided information about a person's emotional states such as anxiety and depression. Eysenck questioned the validity of using psychological descriptions to characterize brain function. He suspected that the brain was more complicated than what was understood at that time.

In opposition to Freud's drive theory, Eysenck published volumes about differences in personality and their biological roots. He showed evidence that emotion is strongly related to the activity of the autonomic nervous system.

In the early 1980s, I recall meeting with a patient, "Harold," who was a 90-year-old retired financial adviser. He was accompanied by his 85-year-old wife, "Judith." During the appointment, I found myself mediating a heated argument between them as Judith was distressed because Harold was seeking daily sexual gratification. He longed for his wife to participate in his sexual fantasies, but Judith adamantly refused.

"His behavior is disgusting, and I want him to stop this nonsense. Tell him it's not natural at his age. Tell him anything, but I can't stand it anymore. I've lived 66 years with this man, and it's enough," she cried.

After listening to her plea, I turned to her husband.

"How can I be of help?" I asked Harold.

"I don't need any help. She does," he replied, pointing his finger at his angry spouse.

Daily sexual activity is unusual for a man of Harold's age, and Judith had a legitimate physical limitation about frequent sexual activity.

"How have you managed your husband's sexual appetite in the past?" I asked her.

"My husband has had a series of women throughout his life. Because he has money, the women found him attractive. Now that he is "over the hill," women don't flock to him like they used to."

After listening to both of them disparage one another, I knew I was in over my head. Within a short period of time, I referred the lively pair to a "couples' therapist." Since Harold did not believe his behavior was abnormal, Judith ended up seeing a psychotherapist on her own.

My experience with EEG/QEEG research has shown that those who constantly seek physical excitation usually need more voltage in the alertness frequencies of the brain. In other words, the brain is trying to wake itself up. Harold's chronic need for sexual stimulation was a clear instance of this.

What I didn't understand at the time was that Harold's unusual sexual appetite - even at his age - was likely driven by his brain's repetitive, automatic impulses to "tune up" or accelerate. Judith had decided that Harold must take care of himself and use his imagination in relieving his physical tensions. Had computerized EEG technology been available in those early years, I might have been helpful to Harold. Unfortunately, this was not the case.

Dr. Richard Caton in Liverpool, England, was the first person to see and record small but constant electrical impulses from the surfaces of living brains in rabbits and monkeys. In 1875, Caton reported to the British Medical Association that he had used a galvanometer to observe electrical impulses.

A half century later, Hans Berger, a Berlin psychiatrist and electro-encephalographic (EEG) pioneer, cited Caton's research in his 1929 report on the discovery of alpha waves. Hans Berger, a German neuropsychiatrist, extracted the first human EEG on his son. He named the dominant electrical activity that he saw alpha waves.

Within five years, EEG machines became available in major medical centers worldwide, and it resulted in rapid medical advances. In the 1930s, neurologists discovered irregular activity in the EEGs of patients suffering with seizures or epilepsy. Without the EEG, doctors could not identify abnormal brain activity.

During this time, neurologists also began to study the brainwaves of healthy adults and noted that each person's visual EEG remained distinct and stable over time.

In 1942, three psychiatric professors in the United States decided to perform a long-term EEG experiment on each other in order to learn how adverse physical challenges would affect their brain electrical activity.

In the beginning, their baseline, eyes closed EEG tracings appeared somewhat similar, but not the same. Then, during the next five years, each professor submitted themselves to brief, stressful challenges, such as sleep deprivation, oxygen deprivation, alcohol poisoning, abdominal bloating, physical fatigue, stomach distension, decompression sickness, low blood sugar, low carbon dioxide exposure, and high doses of an anti-malaria medication.

Each professor's EEG was sampled again during and after each of these stressful events. Two of the professors suffered visual defects and migraine headaches during the stressful events; in addition, their brainwaves distorted into irregular or abnormally slow waves for intervals of time before returning to their usual baseline (awake, alert) EEG pattern.

This experiment showed that visual EEG could track individual brain activity [brainwaves] in real time, during health, medical illness, and restoration of a healthy state.

In the June 1947 issue of *Science,* the doctors reported their findings. They had shown that a person's visual EEG in the resting state is an objective brainwave signature. In addition, they had shown that EEG (sitting, eyes closed) could track a person's brain activity during health, sickness, and restoration of health.

By the mid-twentieth century, EEG pattern recognition suggested the following:

- Baseline brainwaves in healthy adults are individually distinct and stable over time.
- EEG brainwave variations may indicate subtle differences in brain activity.
- EEG technology can track brain activity during health, physical distress, and restoration of health.

Clearly a visual EEG is a characteristic of a person - a brainwave signature; yet, it would take more than 50 years before the value of the EEG as a therapeutic tool would be published.

The development of computers in the 1970s paved the way for pioneering neuroscientists and mathematicians to construct the QEEG, or Quantitative EEG, which is the analysis of the digitized EEG. It is sometimes also called brain mapping. A QEEG device translates the electrical activity of the brain into numbers which are more precise and easier to analyze.

My own research into the benefits of EEG started in 1985. Back then, one of my professors at UCLA suggested that Dr. Steve Suffin and I would make a good professional team and business partners. That suggestion turned out to be prophetic.

Steve was in charge of a psychiatric unit at a local Veterans Administration hospital. Board certified in pathology and psychiatry, Steve was using visual EEG to identify or rule out irregular brainwave activity in psychiatric patients.

We agreed there was an urgent need for a technology that could help us understand the neurophysiology in each patient's psychiatric and/or substance abuse disorder.

During a summer lunch in 1986, Steve and I were discussing the subjective nature of psychiatry and the fact that many patients were not substantially improving. We agreed that the tools we had were insufficient. Steve's father, a general surgeon, overhearing our dissatisfaction, exclaimed, "Why don't you guys go measure something!"

Several months later, Steve and I attended a weekend seminar hosted by Cadwell Laboratories, where we learned about a newly available Neurometrics System of digitized EEG and quantitative EEG (QEEG). It was a safe, painless technology that recorded a person's brainwaves in real time.

QEEG would allow us to record and electronically store a person's brainwaves.

The technology also compared a person's brainwave measures to a database of asymptomatic, physically healthy persons of the same age.

We acquired an EEG/QEEG system in the fall of 1986 and hired a certified EEG technician. We conducted EEGs on ourselves, family members, and interested friends, who said they were asymptomatic. To our relief, none had abnormal or irregular EEG activity, but several had variant QEEG values in the drowsy, alertness, or meditative frequencies. An accomplished, board-certified electro-encephalographer, Dr. Meyer Proler agreed to examine our patients' visual EEGs and identify any irregular or "epileptiform" activity.

By the late 1980s, I had five patients who had suffered for years with symptoms of depression, yet none had improved despite numerous trials of "recommended" antidepressants or anti-anxiety medications or both as suggested by the psychiatric literature. Since each was dysfunctional and demoralized, I asked if they would participate - at no cost - in our clinical EEG/QEEG study.

I would reduce and discontinue their ineffective medication, and they would wait an adequate duration of time until the medications were eliminated from their bodies. Then, my EEG tech would conduct a baseline, un-medicated EEG/QEEG, which I would study in order to develop a physiologic treatment for each patient.

The electro-encephalographer reported that each patient's visual EEG was slightly slow; however, all of them had statistically abnormal QEEG measures in the drowsiness, alertness, and meditative frequencies!

This was a teaching moment! Let me explain.

Similar to a piano, each of these patients' third or fourth octave was tuned too sharp, and (beginning at middle C) the fifth and six octaves were tuned too flat.

Wow! This was complicated and humbling!

But I was relieved because several of these patients had cognitive deficiencies. This confirmed my clinical observation that each of them needed a "tune up" in their alertness frequencies, instead of a tune down.

In other words, the medications I had prescribed using the psychiatric model of linking symptoms and behaviors were not effective. I had been "tuning them down" instead of "tuning them up." That realization explained why they were not improving! From these findings I made the following inferences:

- Unlike medical doctors who use physical data to make a medical diagnosis and select a physical restorative treatment, the DSM is only a behavior sorting system and has no consistent correlation with individual neuro-physiology.

- The DSM system is not a medical diagnostic tool, only a symptomatic and behavioral sorting system.
- No correspondence between symptoms and behaviors and a normalizing medication response exists.

Since medical treatment should improve physiology, what I was doing was not restoring them to a healthy state. Quite the opposite, I didn't seem to be helping them at all. They were still depressed, demoralized, and desperate.

- None of the usual antidepressants recommended by experts had improved their depression.
- The EEG/QEEG showed that the "antidepressants" I had prescribed either had no effect or made them worse.
- These patients needed a brain "tune-up" in their alertness and meditative frequencies, not a "tune-down."
- Both the visual EEG and the QEEG were necessary to understand what each of these patients needed.
- Selecting medications by understanding their biochemical effects in each individual's brain activity was likely to yield a better match and therapeutic outcome.

While my breakthrough treatment dramatically improved the lives of my patients, to their amazement and relief and often within a short time, my journey to arrive at this discovery was far from instant. In fact, my career path would begin in the country's best schools, take me to the world's most dangerous war zones, and land me in sunny Southern California. In the next chapter, we'll explore my personal voyage.

CHAPTER 5

ANIMAL CRACKERS IN MY SOUP/MEDICAL SCHOOL

Coach Norm Lord was better known by his students as "Mr. Clean." The brawny, bald Washington and Lee University (W&L) faculty member had boundless energy. During my freshman year, I was particularly appreciative of his commitment to his students.

At the time, all W&L freshmen were required to run one mile within seven-and- a-half minutes. When I started the university in the fall, I was prepared to take on the academic rigors of my new school. Unfortunately, the timed endurance test wasn't one I could pass. As a result, Mr. Clean provided a training regimen that would elevate my physical fitness to W&L standards.

During the winter months in the state of Virginia, I refused to let the chilly outdoor temperatures stop me. I worked up a sweat running on the indoor track. The following spring, I found myself in the best shape I'd ever been. Up to that point, I'd been more bookish than sporty, but now I had lost excess weight, improved my stamina, and appreciated athletics to the point that I even won a shot-put competition against another college.

The running test was one example among many positive and profound lessons W&L taught me. The strong faculty, academic rigor, interaction with peers from diverse regions of the United States, and the school's hallmark Honor System expanded my thinking and inspired me to grow intellectually.

The Honor System, in particular, made W&L stand out from other universities. It was a code of conduct to maximize trust and minimize lying, cheating, and stealing. Following the Honor System meant that exams were often unsupervised. But the consequences of breaking the Honor System could spell disaster for a student.

I recall a classmate who was caught cheating on a test and another who submitted a research paper peppered with false references. By doing so, both violated the Honor System and were expelled. Sadly, their actions had long-term consequences that cast a shadow on them well beyond their undergraduate years.

In addition, exceptional professors, some eccentric, all brilliant, made it clear why W&L had such an outstanding academic reputation. I still remember, with vivid detail, how Dr. Marshall Fishwick started his European history class:

"Gentlemen, if you want to be rich, don't rob a bank. Steal a country!"

While his lectures were legendary, so were his pop quizzes — cold-sweat-inducing exams where we had to memorize even the footnotes of the readings!

The rigorous memorization required for Dr. Fishwick's class challenged my fact-retention ability. If I were to survive his course, I needed a mnemonic strategy that would keep me academically afloat. By chance, I met a classmate who knew hypnosis. He demonstrated his skill to students in the freshman dorm by hypnotizing volunteers. I gladly played the role of mind-control guinea pig in his displays that were as mesmerizing as Harry Houdini's escape artistry. With repeated practice, I strengthened my concentration and short-term memory. Through the art of self-hypnotism, I learned to tune out exterior noise, which allowed me to excel in Dr. Fishwick's class.

Then there was Dr. James Starling, a senior faculty member in the biology department. He followed up his explanation of nature's unity by encouraging us to "wrap your arms and legs around a tree and say, 'Brother, thee and I are one!'"

But the most memorable professor I had was Dr. Keith Shillington, who taught organic chemistry. Passing the professor's demanding course was a requirement for those, like me, who had medical-school aspirations. Dr. Shillington possessed the power to either open or close the door to a young adult's dream of becoming a medical doctor. Knowing he was the gatekeeper to our professional destiny meant the pressure to succeed in his class was intense.

I can still clearly remember his larger-than-life form, lounging in his wooden chair, scrutinizing his students. As we were painstakingly and silently consumed with our laboratory protocols, he looked on and frequently entertained us with song. His favorite tune? One Shirley Temple sang in the famous 1935 film, *Curly Top*:

Animal crackers in my soup
Monkeys and rabbits loop the loop

Gosh, oh gee, do I have fun
Swallowing animals one by one

While W&L's traditions stood the test of time, not all of them benefited students and the community. During my years there, the university admitted only males to its undergraduate school. Fortunately, the admission of women to its law school in 1972 and to its undergraduate program in 1985 added much-needed feminine yin to the masculine yang.

My long-term goal of becoming a doctor was soon realized when I was accepted to the University of Virginia School (UVA) of Medicine in 1963. Medical school was demanding, yet I was prepared for the academic challenge. UVA and its faculty were world class and left their mark on me.

My present-day bowtie preference stems from my UVA years. The male pediatric faculty chose them over neckties, which infant patients pulled and soiled when physicians leaned forward with a stethoscope to listen to their tiny hearts and lungs.

To spare my parents the burden of medical school tuition, I signed a contract with the US Navy. In exchange for government financial support, I would begin a four-year military service commitment after completing medical school and a one-year internship.

At that time, UVA's psychiatric department stood on oddly unscientific ground. Some of the practices were bizarre. I recall one professor who said he was investigating patients' past lives. I found it strange that he was looking for metaphysical answers to questions unexplained by physical science.

My academic program included a trip to the Western State Hospital in the hills of Virginia. There I witnessed the most pitiful and bizarre remnants of humanity. It reminded me of 18th-century European drawings depicting the mentally insane, minus the chains. Add to these observations my skepticism of widely accepted psychiatric dogma.

The first edition of the *Diagnostic & Statistical Manual of Mental Disorders* (DSM) was published by the American Psychiatric Association in 1952. Although the manual's purpose was (and still is) to organize and categorize symptoms and stigmatizing behaviors, the DSM and its subsequent volumes are intellectually fraudulent.

Rather than being a diagnostic manual, it is only a behavioral sorting system, as acknowledged by the American Psychiatric Association in each version of the DSM. Yet doctors still use this behavioral sorting system for deciding medical treatment. This illogical application would cause Francis Bacon, who described common errors in thinking and misuse of words, to turn over in his grave.

The DSM fallacy of labels vs. measurement is precisely why the psychiatric model is "hard to swallow."

These realizations are some of the reasons I could not imagine at the time pursuing a career in psychiatry. Circumstances, however, would eventually cause me to change my mind.

After four years of medical school at UVA, in 1967, I accepted a one-year surgical internship at Vanderbilt University Medical Center and its associated hospitals in Nashville, Tennessee.

Interns at the medical center were required to rotate through the emergency room at Nashville General Hospital. I'll never forget the grueling 14-to-18-hour shifts, six days a week. Personal time for socializing was rare. My one day off was typically spent relaxing and recovering, preparing for the next demanding six-day cycle.

Within Nashville General Hospital's Emergency Room (ER), I saw injuries so severe that they are forever seared in my memory. Some wounds were a result of carelessness on the patient's part, such as a speed-boat propeller that lodged itself in the skull of an inattentive water skier. Others were due to plain old poor judgment, as with the young man with a ruptured eardrum from a tussle with the police.

Working with colleagues for long periods created a sense of camaraderie and closeness that could sometimes blur the line between professional and personal. I recall becoming attracted to a nursing student. Svetlana had a beautiful face framed by flowing blond hair. One day, after assisting in the surgery of an elderly diabetic patient who had just had his gangrenous lower leg amputated, I spotted Svetlana in the hall. As I was transporting the patient's amputated leg to the pathology lab, I playfully approached her and said, "Hi there! Would you like to see me shake a leg?"

She nodded affirmatively.

Abruptly, I removed the severed limb from its wrapping, lifted it before her eyes, and began shaking the leg in front of her face.

Her horrified response indicated that she was not at all amused by my antics. I immediately regretted what I had done and apologized, explaining it was a sophomoric and inept attempt at flirtation. She gave me a pass for my juvenile behavior, and we maintained a cordial, platonic relationship that lasted through that academic year.

Whether in the operating or emergency room, an intern's work was physically and mentally arduous. As the surgeries became longer in duration, I was compelled to shift weight from one leg to the other in order to reduce an increasing dull ache in my lower back. Over time, these movements were noticeable and annoyed the surgeon. Eventually the increased pain caused me to give up the childhood dream of becoming a surgeon.

After completing my internship in 1968, I began fulfilling my four-year contract with the U.S. Navy, which took me to Da Nang, South Vietnam, in the spring of 1969.

CHAPTER 6

MILITARY SERVICE ABROAD

Once the Continental Airlines passenger door opened, I realized my reality had instantly shifted from the stability of life in the United States to war-torn Vietnam. Repetitive explosions from a near distance penetrated the interior sanctuary of the fuselage. Adrenalin surged in my chest. My skin sprouted goose bumps as I deplaned and descended the stairway to the tarmac below. I kept my eye on the multiple fireballs exploding in the nearby hills. A Jeep was waiting to take me to my new destination, Quang Tri, Vietnam, an abrupt disconnect from Laguna Beach, California.

A few days earlier, I had been a doctor at a naval air station in sunny California, and before that, at Pensacola naval air space in Florida after my internship at Vanderbilt.

Although I could have served most anywhere, I actually enlisted with eight friends volunteering for a tour in Vietnam. Now I was in one of the most dangerous places in the world.

Volunteering to serve in Vietnam was the most daunting challenge I had ever faced. Eventually, unwavering attention to my duties and surroundings would see me through the harrowing events that followed. Yet upon arriving, I felt I had only two options — fear or denial. I initially chose denial and silently affirmed, "Nothing will happen to me."

But no amount of denial could diminish the sound of repetitive explosions followed by bursts of black smoke in the surrounding distant grassy hills as I walked over the tarmac to the Huey gunship helicopter ready to fly me to Quang Tri. Harsh wartime conditions would not keep me from accepting my new reality.

I was the new flight surgeon for Helicopter Squadron HMM-262. By the time I arrived, what would become the historic Tet Offensive in that region had ended with severe casualties and losses on both the American and North Vietnamese sides.

Quang Tri airbase was one of the most dangerous locations in Vietnam. Garbed in black during the night, the Viet Cong were as persistent as cockroaches, trying to penetrate the perimeter fence and enter the airbase. Unbeknown to us, one of them was eventually identified as our squadron's barber and could easily have slit our throats.

I shared a Quonset hut — or hooch in military slang — with seven pilots. My living area was a 5-by-10-foot space at one end of the structure. At night, we heard the ear-piercing screams of approaching rockets. John Whitworth, a pilot in our squadron, and I excavated a small space outside our end of the hooch and fortified it with cinderblocks. It was wishful thinking that it provided protection. I became occupied with listening for rockets and observing fleeting patches of landscape as our flares illuminated the sky above the airbase's perimeter. Gradually, I became less reactive to the incoming rockets.

HMM-262 pilots flew the CH-46, a twin-rotor helicopter that was built to transport troops in and out of battle zones and conduct medical evacuations. Occasionally, I flew on these medical evacuation missions. Flight surgeons were not encouraged to fly, as they were not easily replaced, but I sensed an ethical bond with the corpsmen. What Marine helicopter pilots, crewmen, and navy corpsmen accomplished was often miraculous.

Within minutes, we could transform the elongated cabin of a CH-46 into a flying emergency room. The most important mission was to recover the dead and wounded. If we could transport a wounded marine within 30 minutes to Charlie Med, a field hospital eight miles away, he was likely to survive.

About a decade later, during the early years of psychiatric medical practice, my administrator called during an interlude between patients.

"Dr. Emory, a young man who says he was a Marine in Vietnam just walked into the reception room. He says you saved his life in Vietnam and wants to thank you."

A moment later, the Marine veteran, in his late twenties, appeared in my office and expressed his appreciation for my saving his life. He had researched the HMM-262 squadron's flight log to identify the pilots, medical corpsman, and doctor who had treated him during his flight to Charlie Med nearly a decade earlier. I did not recognize him, but I did recall a visual memory of that frantic flight.

Eight wounded Marines had been rushed onto the floor of the helicopter. We had no time to waste! Our immediate task was to assure an airway, minimize bleeding, and keep them alive. The Marine who stood before me must have been one of them.

I thanked the young man for finding me and for his expression of gratitude. It was a reflection of his good character and consistent with the Marine Corps motto, "Semper Fidelis" (always faithful).

After military duty with the First Marine Aircraft Wing in Vietnam, in 1970, I was assigned to the U.S. Naval Air Facility at Sigonella, located near Catania, Sicily. I was there until 1972.

At the time, the hospital was a small medical facility with outpatient, inpatient, and emergency services for active duty navy personnel and their families. Whether diagnosing and treating a patient with a urinary tract infection, with a painful kidney stone, or with injuries from an accident on the base, the hospital emergency facilities were equipped to handle whatever emergencies might arise.

Shortly after I arrived at Sigonella, an auto accident occurred near the air facility, and soon thereafter, an injured young man who worked at the Naval base was brought into the emergency room.

He was severely short of breath and suffering with a heart rate over a hundred beats per minute — extremely abnormal considering that 65 to 80 is typical for a healthy adult. A chest X-ray showed three fractured left ribs and a collapsed left lung. This injury was an emergency! He needed a chest tube to expand his collapsed left lung and restore the ability to adequately oxygenate his blood.

After inserting the chest tube, his heart rate and breathing normalized.

Several days later, five men dressed in grey overcoats and Italian fedoras appeared in my office requesting to see me. To my surprise, I was staring into the face of the Mafia chief of Eastern Sicily.

In Italian he said, "The man whose life you saved two nights ago is my brother. I came to thank you. If there is anything we can do for you, don't hesitate to ask."

I was surprised and somewhat numb from sleep deprivation but cautiously responded, "There is something you can do for me. Several days ago, while I was shopping in Catania, someone broke into my car and stole several new suits and groceries, including the Sara Lee Cheesecakes, which are the favorite among my Italian friends."

The capo de Mafiosi requested, in Italian,

"Give me the day, time, and street address where you parked your car."

My response was quick and to the point. Nodding in my direction, the Mafia chief turned to his associates and left without another word.

A few days later, the hospital administrator informed me that my suits had just been returned. Unfortunately, the groceries, including the cheesecakes, were not recovered. I learned that the suits had been sent to the city of Syracuse, 43 miles away, and were recovered in an apparel shop!

Later that day, I received a phone call from the Mafia chief who repeated, "If there is anything else we can do for you, Doctor, don't hesitate to ask." At this point, I had sufficient sense not to make a further request, although I wished they had returned my beloved dessert as well.

Decades later, my role as a doctor would connect me with yet another criminal family, this time on U.S. soil. I provided expert testimony at what eventually became one of the most high-profile trials of the last century.

On November 3, 1993, I was to testify in the case of Lyle and Erik Menendez in the murder of their parents, Kitty and José Menendez. A year earlier, Mrs. Menendez had overdosed on medication and had been admitted to the Westlake Medical Center. As the director of the Medical Stress Unit, I was asked to complete a psychiatric medical assessment on Mrs. Menendez. I concluded that she was highly distressed, vulnerable, and warranted being transferred to the local psychiatric hospital. However, when her husband appeared and refused my advice, she was immediately discharged. Because of my connection to Mrs. Menendez, the court requested my testimony.

The day before my scheduled appearance in court, I was seeing patients at my Thousand Oaks office when I was abruptly interrupted with an urgent message: Much of Malibu was ablaze, and strong winds were directing the fire toward my neighborhood and my house. A major downside of living in one of the world's most spectacular locations is its susceptibility to natural disasters. That day, my neighborhood was being evacuated.

Immediately, I drove home to assess the situation. Ominous black smoke covered the sky as the fire devoured hillside homes in its race toward the ocean. As I entered my neighborhood adjacent to the beach, a mass of fire trucks, firefighters, and police were ordering residents to evacuate. People were fleeing one way or another via the Pacific Coast Highway. The major road to and out of the area was chaotic, filled with fire trucks entering from other municipalities to fight the blaze and residents leaving Malibu in both directions along the way.

I had about 40 minutes before the roads would be closed to everyone. I showed my driver's license to the police, and they informed me that residents had no time to waste.

Once home, I grabbed some suitcases, collected family albums, videos, documents, my computer, and clothing, filling two cars to the brim. Then, realizing that I had to drive both cars down a steep hill and out of Malibu, I donned a pair of track shoes. The strategy was to drive each vehicle down to the Pacific Coast highway and out of the fire zone. Despite my long-distance training, executing the plan was challenging.

After performing this back-and-forth maneuver for a couple of miles, a friend from the city suddenly appeared on his bicycle and offered to assist in the evacuation. Was I happy to see him! We dissembled his bike and placed it in one car. Then I ran back to the second car, and we drove toward the city, away from the smoke that was enveloping Malibu. I learned several days later, my home and many others were destroyed, but fortunately no lives were lost.

I spent that evening with friends in Westwood, and the next morning drove to the Van Nuys Federal Court to testify in the Menendez trial. Having lost most of my belongings, I looked as though I had been through the wringer. And I had! I pride myself on being a well-dressed person at all times, and to my chagrin, outside the courtroom, I found myself sitting next to two internationally known, well-dressed authors. I suddenly realized this event might be the trial of the century, and here I was in crumpled attire, an unprofessional image that could negatively affect the perception of my testimony.

After waiting for what seemed like an eternity, I was called into the courtroom and sworn in, now in front of the judge, prosecutors, and defense team. Having been informed about my circumstance, the presiding judge pounded his gavel and said, "Off the record! Ladies and gentlemen, Dr. Hamlin Emory is here to testify this morning, despite the loss of his home in yesterday's Malibu fire. Thank you, Dr. Emory. Now, back on the record!" as he struck the gavel again and continued the proceedings.

CHAPTER 7

DEVELOPING A NEW PATIENT-TREATMENT PARADIGM

Reflecting on my military experience, I recall working as a general medical doctor at Camp Pendleton in Southern California prior to being flown off to Vietnam. One afternoon, a Marine Corps sergeant trudged into the dispensary hallway and stood before me with erect, military posture and a stoic face.

"Doc, I need your help," he told me.

"Come into my office, Sergeant," I replied.

Closing the door, he limped across the room and sat on the exam table. His facial expression soon transformed, suggesting profound suffering. I noted his ashen face and bloodshot eyes. Suddenly the soldier burst into tears.

"What's wrong?" I asked.

Without a word and with great difficulty, the sergeant removed his boots, displaying an infected foot and lower leg. He had a serious case of cellulitis, which is an infection that, in his case, had progressed nearly to his knee and needed immediate medical treatment. This simple example from my general medical experience shows how medical illnesses can be external, visible, and obvious. But what if the illness is internal and not apparent? This kind of condition is more challenging.

As a trained physician, external conditions, such as this solder's infected foot, are easier to treat because a doctor can see them. Internal disorders, which some doctors may loosely label by a patient's symptoms and behaviors, are more challenging because they are not detectable by visual inspection or lab tests.

The psychiatric model has not and still does not identify the neurophysiologic variations that cause chronic brain-based mental disorders.

Healthy persons enjoy predictable physical and mental wellbeing. Yet those with chronic mental disorders or substance abuse do not have such capacity. This fact explains why persons with brain-based mental disorders find ways to relieve the agony of their abnormal neurobiology. Persistent substance abuse, bingeing, purging, restricting food obsession, compulsions, self-mutilation, outward aggression, violence, and more are behaviors that temporarily improve neurophysiology.

Without a comprehensive medical approach that includes measurement of individual neurophysiology, doctors and healthcare professional assumptions may not be correct.

Despite initially being convinced that psychiatry wasn't for me when I was a student at UVA, I eventually changed my mind.

With my tour in Italy coming to an end, I began my residency program at the Veteran's Hospital in West Los Angeles. My next stop was the UCLA Campus just steps away.

Unlike my training in medical school and at Vanderbilt Medical Center, psychiatric residency at UCLA taught doctors to use symptoms and maladaptive behaviors as medical diagnoses without physical measurement. Patients were usually prescribed antipsychotic, antidepressant, or anti-anxiety medications, all of which often caused tremors, similar to Parkinson's disease, and other side effects. Many were hospitalized because of the negative effects of these powerful drugs. The goal was to find another medication that decreased the tremors. I conformed to the psychiatric approach. Although I did not physically examine my patients, I tried to understand their invisible illness through the power of words in psychotherapy. In many cases, talk therapy proved ineffective.

I soon realized that while my professors and fellow residents were intelligent — even brilliant — they violated the medical model by adopting terms from the psychological theorists in an attempt to treat problematic symptoms, thoughts, and behavior.

No psychiatric professor that I recall ever monitored patients' abnormal physical findings. Rather, the focus was on psycho-social interactions. We claimed to be treating brain disorders but lacked a way to measure them. Instead, we guessed about what medication to prescribe for individual neurobiology.

During my first year at UCLA's Neuropsychiatric Institute, I was assigned responsibility for "Albert," a young adult male with a graduate school degree.

A few years earlier, he had the onset and then progression of episodic rage, was labeled a paranoid schizophrenic, and was prescribed an antipsychotic medication that was sedating but also causing adverse effects such that he was unable to continue his employment.

Reviewing his physical systems, a standard practice I learned in medical school, I asked, "Do you experience any unusual sensations in your body before the episodes of irritability, anger, or rage?"

"Yes," he said.

The medical literature in the 1950s had described clinical differences between schizophrenia and temporal lobe epilepsy, and his answer suggested he was suffering from temporal lobe epilepsy, not schizophrenia. But no clinician had previously asked this question. So, I ordered an electroencephalogram (EEG), which is a visual analysis of a person's brainwave activity.

The neurology professor's EEG report noted recurrent, abnormal electrical brain activity in both temporal lobes that was interfering with his regular brainwaves. The diagnosis was, as I had suspected, temporal lobe epilepsy. Had I not made this discovery, who knows how long the patient would have suffered under a misdiagnosis — perhaps for his entire life.

It was clear that this young man had been mis-medicated for two years and required an immediate change in prescription. I converted him from the antipsychotic to an anticonvulsant and dosed it in a low-normal range. He experienced no negative effects. Within two months, he became healthy again and returned to his prior employment — without a trace of his so-called schizophrenia. For over a decade after treatment, he sent me a thank-you note on the anniversary of his return to sanity.

During my psychiatric residency, physical examination of patients was not emphasized. If patients were physically ill, they were referred to another department. Years later, my research lead me to understand why this approach was difficult for me to accept fully.

In 1976, after completing UCLA's psychiatric residency program, I began a traditional psychiatric practice treating children, adolescents, and adults at several suburban Los Angeles hospitals. After a number of years, I decided to practice in Thousand Oaks, California.

At the time, Thousand Oaks was the "Wild West," with very few practitioners. I recall the day I phoned my mother back in the state of Virginia to let her know I was going to make California my professional home.

I noted that a number of my patients had physical ailments, such as learning problems, high blood pressure, fast pulse rates, and migraine headaches. As taught in my residency program, I referred them to other medical specialists. Yet the results were often not satisfactory. Over time, what began as frustration on my part turned into curiosity.

One patient in particular propelled me into taking more effective action. 'Larry' had been diagnosed as a manic depressive and was prescribed lithium by another physician. Lithium is widely used as a mood stabilizer; however, Larry's mood remained unstable. For a number of weeks, I conducted psychotherapy, only to find no improvement to his mood.

Sensing a professional obligation to ameliorate his condition, I realized I had reached a crossroads: Either apply the medical model to patients with disordered behavior or follow the psychiatric guidelines, and abstain from using the medical model, and severely limit my patients.

I soon retrieved my medical bag that I had set aside years ago. It held my physical exam tools — my blood pressure cuff and stethoscope — I hoped to do better. I hired a nurse and once again, as in years before, began to physically examine my patients and monitor their vital signs, height, weight, and body mass index.

My decision to employ medical practices with psychiatric treatments signaled the start of a journey that would eventually span nearly four decades, where I learned how to identify, classify, and improve variations in brain function.

I began to monitor Larry's vital signs over the course of several days. I discovered he had a chronically fast pulse rate, which prompted me to prescribe a beta blocker, reducing the excessive adrenalin in his body. The results were outstanding. His pulse and blood pressure normalized, and his mood stabilized. Larry was no longer a manic depressive because medically he had never been one in the first place.

Today, prescribing medications following standard psychiatric guidelines provides questionable results. In fact, adverse reactions from the psychiatric approach cause nearly 90,000 adult emergency room visits in the United States every year, including accidental overdoses, and almost one in five results in hospitalization. With evidence like this, the current psychiatric treatment model clearly has room for improvement. In my opinion it is, for the most part, just guessing.

Observing the misery of hospitalized psychiatric patients in the 1980s and 1990s was repugnant. Most were overly tranquilized. Cognitive dulling, despair, anxiety, and adverse medication effects were the negative physical outcomes. Unlike my experience in general medical practice, my colleagues and I were merely making a significant percent of patients "less worse." Psychiatric labels were not correlating with medication response.

In the 1980s, while in private practice, I recognized that my colleagues and I had no objective means to make distinctions in the neurobiology of each patient — we treated symptoms and behaviors with no thought about the differences in individual brain function. Jerome Groopman, MD, said it well in 2007 when he wrote, "Doctors learn by their mistakes on live patients." My psychiatric colleagues and I had no objective way of doing that because we had no observable information about each patient's biology or neurophysiology.

Even worse, I was prescribing medication using trial and error without knowing how each medication affected a patient's brain activity. I could only determine if I made them better or worse by listening to their subjective report and by observing their behavior. I could only observe whether the medication had adverse effects. At best, most of my patients achieved a reduction of symptoms with some improvement in functionality.

Unlike my experience in surgical training and clinical medicine, only a small percent of people whom I treated actually became well. Most of the time, I was merely applying mental Band-Aids.

My training at the Veterans Hospital and UCLA's Neuropsychiatric Institute emphasized evaluating the cognition of every patient; however, most patients referred to me had not had a thorough cognitive exam. I was reminded of Lord Campbell's quote:

"Until you take what you do and express it in numbers, your knowledge of it is of a meager and unsatisfactory sort."

The brain is the supreme organ, and how well it functions determines the course of one's life! As I struggled with the disillusionment and frustration of trying to improve the treatment of patients, I also began to read and study the great thinkers of the recent and more distant past. William Osler (1849-1919) was one of the most admired academic medical professors in the history of modern medicine. In addition, I revisited Aristotle and his works to immerse myself in the study of the validity of knowledge. Francis Bacon, the person who clearly defined the limitations of inductive reasoning, was another great thinker whose work was of great interest to me. The following case studies emphasize the result of my journey and a new patient paradigm.

CHAPTER 8

TORTURED IN A SEA OF ADRENALIN

A decade ago, a man stood before me, looking as if he had just escaped from an electrocution. Hair blown asunder, unshaven, overweight, terrified, he blurted, "I was in the ER this morning! They gave me an injection of something to calm me. Then I was told to take a pill three times a day. Doc, I don't have a normal life with this illness."

It was as if "Ivan the Terrible" were torturing him, but the tormentor was his own body.

"Marcus" had been an A student from elementary through graduate schools. At that time, he had been highly functional in a competitive profession. However, increasing alcohol consumption had rendered him disabled, unemployable, and dependent on Social Security.

"I pace all night and am desperate for relief," he told me. His blood pressure and pulse rates were dangerously high.

"I want to function like I used to, but this anxiety kills the drive I used to have. For God's sake, can you help me?" he asked.

He had four years of consultations with several psychiatrists. Their treatment included antidepressants, antipsychotics and anticonvulsants, which caused sedation. Drug cocktails like these are common in psychiatric prescribing. Such attempts are mostly temporary efforts to alleviate symptoms and often lead to "stacking" medications.

These treatments proved ineffective and caused Marcus to gain 45 pounds, lose his libido and render him unable to continue his profession. In addition, he became alienated from family and friends.

His health deteriorated. Desperate and demoralized, he was admitted to an emergency room where he was prescribed tranquilizers. He was terrified. His facial expression reminded me of how I felt during a medevac mission in Vietnam when the pilot announced that we were landing in a hot zone to take on casualties. That moment of fear was this man's daily life.

Clinical research had taught me why Marcus found comfort in daily doses of alcohol and marijuana. My task as his doctor was to convert his suffering into neurophysiologic reasoning. After performing a physical exam, I concluded that this brilliant man had inherited a condition associated with excessive adrenalin. This excess caused his pulse and blood pressure to soar. After consulting with his cardiologist, I prescribed a medication that reduced his excessive adrenalin.

Marcus's pulse and blood pressure normalized within a few hours. He returned to my office the following week and happily announced, "Doc, my pulse is now 68 and I'm not so nervous. I sleep better and don't pace like I used to." His smile was contagious.

"Does anyone else observe your improvement?" I asked.

"Yes, my family says they actually like me."

CHAPTER 9

LEFT FOR DEAD

One Saturday afternoon, my wife and I were window shopping in Beverly Hills when my cell phone buzzed. I recognized the caller's number from Washington state.

"Hello, Bob."

"Hi, Hamlin. We have a problem with 'Malia,' a six-year-old girl in our Kenyan orphanage. She's losing weight and has repetitive seizures that increase each day.

Malia had a horrific start in life. Her mother had squatted in a field, gave birth to her and walked away. Shortly thereafter, a passerby found her near death and brought her to the orphanage run by Bob's Christian charity. Malia had repetitive seizures and was being treated with an antiseizure medication. However, this treatment worsened her condition. Bob was desperate for my help.

"Hamlin, do you have any recommendations?" he asked.

I knew that excessive slow brain activity can increase the risk of seizures.

"Bob, aspirin accelerates brain electrical activity, and we can use it as a quick probe to decide how to help her. If you have children's aspirin at the orphanage, give it to her twice a day and call me tomorrow with an update."

Bob phoned me the next day, and as I had hoped, the seizures had decreased in frequency. Despite this positive outcome, I cautioned Bob that aspirin was only a temporary measure. To develop a long-term treatment plan, an EEG would be necessary.

Fortunately, the staff at the orphanage was able to drive Malia 60 miles to the nearest hospital. Within a short period of time, an EEG was performed and electronically transferred to my laboratory in Los Angeles. The results were not a surprise.

Malia's sitting pulse rates were excessively fast, and her brain waves were slow. I knew we needed to

- first, lower her dose of antiseizure medication in order to speed up her brain waves;
- second, prescribe clonidine, which would reduce her fast pulse rate; and
- third, add Ritalin to accelerate her alertness frequencies.

I explained, "Bob, here is a metaphor that you can convey to the nurse. If Malia were a light bulb, this treatment will make her a brighter and cooler bulb." Over the years I have learned that an important order in prescribing medications, is necessary. I treat the fast waves before the slow waves and the high voltages before the low. If this order is not followed, the outcomes are poor.

For the last eight years, this treatment has normalized her fast pulse rate, increased her alertness and improved her ability to function socially and academically.

Thanks to the EEG data, I was able to improve the health of a six-year-old child whom I have never seen and is living on the other side of the world.

CHAPTER 10

A LIFE WORTH LIVING

"Doctor, I've been a sober member of the 12 -step program for almost 35 years. I have seen countless psychiatrists and psychologists and been in a number of treatment centers for substance abuse. Today I'm celebrating a clean life of 15 years."

This was "Claude's" introductory statement to me when I first met him.

He went on to describe the nature of his IV-drug addiction: being diagnosed with Hepatitis C. "Hey, Doc, I have been in some pretty bad places, but the worst was when I was diagnosed with Hepatitis C. As an IV-drug user, I watched friends suffer through the treatment. Some died."

After taking Methadone and Interferon and experiencing horrible withdrawals, he stopped taking the medications his previous doctor had prescribed. His resistance to taking medication recommended by his physician came from years of bias at Alcoholics Anonymous (AA) and Narcotics Anonymous (NA). These programs ingrained within him false notions that any substances, even those designed to treat his substance abuse and depression, would cause him great harm. He declared, "All drugs are bad, and anyone who takes them will regret they ever started." He believed drugs led to mental illness, incarceration, and death.

But when Claude's liver began shutting down, he decided to follow his doctor's advice. Given his skepticism for the medical establishment and the advice it dispensed, I asked what led him to contact me.

"I imagined being balanced — that means not smoking two packs of cigarettes a day, eating pints of ice cream at night to sleep, gaining weight, and hating myself even more. The Hep-C kept me from having sex. You know, doc, I'm an honorable guy at the core. So rather than disclose my disease before having sex, I decided to avoid sex altogether. For a long time, I didn't tell anyone about the disease because I carried a deep sense of shame and guilt; it felt like a big metal shackle around my ankle, like the ones inmates wear. The Hep-C was the last remnant of what I had done to myself."

Claude explained that he sought me out to verify through tests that he had an imbalance within his brain function. He pointed to his head and said, "I want proof there's something wrong here."

Years before, he bought a *Physicians Desk Reference* so he could tell the doctors what his symptoms were in order to get the drugs he wanted. He knew the Hep-C treatment could cause cancer and liver damage. Since his immunity was already poor, his sponsor gave him the okay to proceed with treatment. In spite of the OK from his sponsor, Claude was scared.

"What if you find a piece of my brain missing? I'm taking a big risk by seeing you," he said.

Opiates gave him energy and a certain calmness that made him feel better. Now I am telling him that his brain function could improve without opiates.

I agreed with the basic tenets of popular recovery programs, including AA and NA. But what is often missing in these approaches is attending to brain activity and, specifically, moving from sub-optimal to optimal brain function. Merging neuroscience with AA principles is an effective combination.

After performing my assessment, I determined he needed to begin taking two types of medication. One would energize him while the other would calm him. The medication prescribed would tune up frequencies associated with awake, alert and calm. I explained to Claude that, "This medication is food for your brain."

One benefit of his Alcoholics and Narcotic Anonymous background was that it gave him an appreciation for the role a sponsor played in his recovery. He regarded me as his medical sponsor, and thus closely followed my recommendations. Unfortunately, many members of his recovery program disapproved of our treatment plan. But Claude knew his options were limited, and he was desperate to make dramatic changes in order to improve his life.

He was fearful of becoming bedridden and going through his life savings in six months of treatment. After eight weeks of following my plan, we retested him using EEG/QEEG. For him, the results were nothing short of miraculous. His brain function had normalized. In addition, he stopped feeling sick as he went through his Hepatitis C treatment. In fact, he was able to work and resume exercise.

"I'm alive, Doc! I'm still alive!" he told me after I had given him the results of his follow-up EEG/QEEG.

Through our work together, Claude eventually understood that the deadly diseases we call alcoholism and drug addiction are often the result of resourceful people self medicating an inherited imbalance in their brain function.

"The few people who were my friends are no longer my friends. After nine months, I'm functioning better than ever. The Hep-C treatment is behind me, and I'm virus free. I have energy, a sex drive, and I sleep at night. All this without pain medication!"

Claude continues to attend AA and NA meetings and has a sponsor. The difference now is he realizes he needs to feel well in order to stay sober. Claude is like so many others who abuse substances because they don't feel well when they are sober.

"All the meetings in the world and all the steps, a thousand times over, would not give me the healthy body I have now. Maybe one day someone will open a rehab center where each person's brain is treated along with the 12 steps program. I pray that will happen soon. I finally have a life worth living."

CHAPTER 11

I THOUGHT I WAS JUST A JERK

"Dr. Emory, our son 'Andrew,' developed abilities earlier than his peers. He did well until high school and then became anxious and moody. We spent six years and thousands of dollars on psychiatrists and therapists. The last doctor labeled him with bipolar disorder and prescribed a seizure medicine with lithium. It makes him slow, but he says his thoughts are racing."

Andrew's parents were worried and desperate. There was no history of mental illness in either family. Their son had reported onset of low moods in high school and had medicated himself with drugs and alcohol. His symptoms worsened in college, so he consulted a psychiatrist and was prescribed a series of SSRI antidepressants (selective serotonin reuptake inhibitors) and an antipsychotic medication.

The parents lamented, "These medicines are not working, and they are now calling Andrew bipolar. He's on a benzodiazepine tranquilizer, and now taking more than originally prescribed." (Benzodiazepines shift the EEG spectrum faster), therefore, they can be normative with some people who have an anxiety, mood and/or an attentional difficulty. "Then the doctor was worried, took him off the benzo and replaced it with another anticonvulsant that slows him down. Now he is a zombie, feeling worse than ever before. He just withdrew from college, and that's why we are here."

Andrew was a fine-looking 23-year-old sitting in my consultation room. Since he was not an athlete, his persistently low blood pressure (101/60) and pulse (59) were significant physical findings. Psychologically, he was sad, and his inability to do simple mathematics was extremely abnormal.

After the initial consultation and baseline (unmedicated) EEG/QEEG, it was clear to me Andrew needed a "tuning up." When I prescribed Dexedrine at a moderate dose, his cognitive ability normalized. Simple math was no longer difficult for him. His mood lifted noticeably, and after a year on this compound, he asked me if he could wean himself off the medicine. He understood the importance of maintaining his much-improved brain wave activity yet wanted a more natural approach. I suggested he try replacing the Dexedrine with an amino acid precursor of dopamine.

His parents were pleased with that decision yet were concerned about their son's emotional health. Would he slip back into melancholy? Would he be okay on just an amino acid? Well, the good news is that Andrew did just fine on the amino acid because he took enough of them to mimic a weak Dexedrine. To his parents' delight, Andrew was soon able to pursue his professional career.

CHAPTER 12

I CAN'T STOP PULLING OUT MY HAIR

"Helen," a well-dressed middle-aged professional woman, sat before me in my office. As she described her distress, I noticed several balding areas on her scalp that concerned me. She had been prescribed numerous brain-slowing medications that psychiatrists use for this symptom. Her weight was average, and her pulse and blood pressure were low for her age.

I asked," What happens just before you begin to pull out your hair?"

Her reply was, "I have the sensation that's like a tickle. The only way to relieve it is to pull out my hair."

"When you pull out your hair, how do you feel?"

"I'm relieved for a while, but then this sensation comes back throughout the day. Then, I have to pull at my hair once more, just to get more relief. It's driving me crazy!"

I noted there was no hair pulling when she was speaking with me.

Her EEG/ QEEG voltages were low across all brain regions. This result informed me that she would not likely improve with customary antidepressant/anti-anxiety medications. Her alertness frequencies needed to be powered up, not slowed down.

Experience taught me that she needed one of the most voltage accelerating medications available, a MAO inhibitor. This class of medication can increase the blood pressure and pulse rate. For this reason there is a risk in prescribing this kind of medication, unless the doctor has comprehensive physical and neurological data which includes EEG/QEEG measurement. Helen's EEG measurements informed me that this would likely be the normalizing choice for her brain activity.

Six months later, Helen burst into my office and said, "Doctor Emory, look at my hair. It's thick and curly. I can't remember having hair like this since I was 10 years old. I am no longer ashamed of my natural hair and no longer wear a wig."

CHAPTER 13

YOU'RE TOO EMOTIONAL!

In the early 2000s, "Victoria," an attractive older woman, sat in my consultation room, captivating my interest with an unusual history. More than 50 years earlier, as a five-year-old, she sat in a hospital hallway with her mother, awaiting blood tests after a recent strep throat infection. Peering through an operating room doorway, Victoria witnessed a tiny newborn being lifted feet first from a cold white table. The doctor was holding a large hypodermic needle, ready to thrust it into the tiny skull of the infant. Immediately, she panicked, screaming in horror, "Mommy, look at that!"

"My mother tried to distract me by standing in front of the open doorway, but I still hear the squealing sounds of protestation from the baby. I held my ears, but the sound became unbearable, and then I fainted."

Young Victoria lapsed into unconsciousness, striking her head on the concrete floor. It was the first of many fainting episodes she would experience.

After an x-ray ruled out a skull fracture, she and her mother returned home. This frightening experience established a deep-seated phobia of blood and needles. At age seven, while showing her father a bloody loose tooth, she passed out again, striking her head on the rim of the bathtub.

Such episodes increased in frequency. At age nine, Victoria was subjected to a series of EEGs. Despite repeated testing, the results were always reported as "normal," and yet, Victoria continued to faint.

Moving forward through adolescence, the next major event happened at 16, in a health class as she watched a film depicting children about to receive their annual inoculations. That was all it took to send alarm bells ringing in her ears. She immediately alerted her football star classmate, whispering, "Alex, I'm about to faint. Don't be scared." And so, she did, collapsing on top of him.

"The next thing I knew, the teacher was peering over me as I lay on the floor. Utterly embarrassed, I struggled to my feet, only to fall again. Alex carefully lifted and escorted me to the school nurse's office. That incident bonded us for the next four years."

Victoria was a compulsive consumer of sweets, especially dark chocolate. The result was frequent cavities and dental appointments. Once there, she made it clear that no Novocain was to be used saying, "I'm more afraid of needles than pain."

I asked if her neurologists had considered a seizure disorder. She insisted that her physicians had ruled out this possibility. Fifty-five years of testing had found no irregular mental or neurological abnormalities. "I'm just emotional," she said. "The doctors' remedy for my concerns is, don't get upset."

As a young housewife in her mid-20s, a movie date with her husband turned alarming when a bloody movie scene led to another fainting episode. Her physician husband, observing her eyes involuntarily diverting to the right, knew she was having a seizure. But what was there to do? Regardless of what numerous neurologists told her, it became increasingly evident that Victoria was suffering from an unidentified illness.

As years passed, her seizures grew more intense, causing her limbs to stiffen with each episode. After two hospitalizations and routine neurological examinations, the neurologists insisted that Victoria exhibited no signs of abnormal brainwave activity. Once again, her complaints were dismissed.

At age 46, during a weekend in Palm Springs, while lying down watching TV, Victoria felt dizzy. Anticipating this was a prelude to another fainting episode, she raced into the bedroom and threw herself on the bed with her head over the side, as her husband watched in horror.

"Hold me down," she muttered. "This is going to be a bad one." Gaining consciousness, her husband told her she experienced a grand mal seizure. "But I knew it wasn't over as two more grand mal seizures followed in quick succession."

Paramedics brought her to the ER, where a CT scan ruled out a brain tumor. The doctor administered an IV containing anti-seizure medication, which caused her to feel nauseated and even more dizzy. She groaned as the medication coursed through her body. After begging the physicians to remove the IV, she was prescribed additional "antiepileptic" medication. Once at home, Victoria threw the pills in the garbage.

After the ER doctor in Palm Springs reported Victoria's case to the DMV, her driver's license was suspended for six months. Dependent on neighbors to transport her children to and from school, she became obsessively fearful of losing consciousness in public, and avoided leaving her home. It was a year before she felt comfortable driving the family car.

I explained that most anti-seizure medications reduce alertness and increase drowsiness.

"No wonder I'm tired all the time!" she exclaimed.

I asked if her doctors suggested any other treatment.

"They told me my problem was psychological, and psychotherapy was the treatment of choice. After 25 years of analysis, I am still in the same predicament as before. Can you imagine?"

At 61 years of age and desperate to find an answer to her dilemma, Victoria heard about my medical approach, and the use of EEG/QEEG to improve brain activity. During the initial consult, her sitting pulse rates were abnormally low. Despite her education and intelligence, she had difficulty subtracting a series of numbers, and her immediate recall of a brief paragraph was deficient, causing me to suspect a variance in brain function.

Though her visual EEG showed no abnormal activity, quantification of her brainwaves (QEEG) showed low voltages (power) across all areas of her brain in frequencies associated with alertness. These findings were consistent with her history of chronic fatigue, lack of attention to detail, and an insatiable appetite for sweets. Victoria's appetite for sweets was excessive, craving and consuming it day and night. As a child she used her weekly allowance to buy candy at the local drug store. The result was, she had little appetite at mealtimes. She even hid the candy in her closet. When her mother cleaned her room and found the hidden candy wrappers, she raised her hands in horror.

Her medical history and physical and cognitive findings, as well as her EEG/QEEG measures, showed that she required speeding up of her alertness frequencies. Today, Victoria reports increased energy and less craving for candy or chocolate on this regimen.

Her brainwave signature informed me that her physical and psychological health would only improve by increasing her voltages across all areas of her brain. The anti-seizure medications her neurologists had previously prescribed, had done the opposite, causing a physician induced illness! This is common in everyday medicine across all medical specialties.

Once prescribed a medication that increased her dopamine, Victoria experienced a more satisfying solution, and her craving for sweets were markedly reduced. Another effect was less cavities.

Numerous follow-up EEG/QEEGs over ensuing years show that her brain electrical activity has increased to within normal limits. It has been more than 15 years since Victoria fainted or had a seizure.

CHAPTER 14

LOOKING BEYOND SYMPTOMS AND BEHAVIORS

In 1937, Kurt Lewin, the founder of social psychology, wrote a book in which he stated, "The oscillation of a pendulum, the falling of an apple from a tree and rolling of the stone down an inclined plane — each of these phenotypes looks quite different, but each is the product of the laws of gravity." Lewin was cautioning psychologists to think about the possibility that people with different behaviors might have similar brain function. In addition, patients with different physical abnormalities can have similar symptomology. Therefore, it is necessary to look beyond symptoms and behaviors to the actual brain variance that is causing the patient's distress.

"Henry" was referred to me following his discharge from a local psychiatric hospital. He had been diagnosed and treated as a schizophrenic patient. While conducting a physical examination, I discovered that he had a constantly fast pulse rate, a physical abnormality, that had not been identified by the hospital doctor. Henry had been misdi-agnosed. Although his visual EEG was normal, two abnor-mal features in the QEEG were apparent. The fast pulse rate had to be addressed first. This treatment required an adrenalin-reducing beta blocker. The second agent was an amphetamine to improve his alertness frequencies. This is the opposite of what you would expect. Combined with the adrenalin reducing agent, the amphetamine converted Henry into brain-body balance. For him it was a normal-izing experience. Within a short period of time, Henry was able to return to the university and successfully complete his education.

This patient was one of many misdiagnosed individuals with a persistently fast pulse rate. The abnormal pulse rate had not been identified by other physicians. Such patients require a thorough monitoring of blood pressure and pulse rates, along with a physical examination and a technology that can inform their doctor how to improve their brain function. EEG/QEEG is the least invasive technology to assist doctors in making this pivotal decision.

CHAPTER 15

KILL YOURSELF

"My daughter, 'Gabriela,' had straight A's in school and played in the high school orchestra until recently. She has difficulty sleeping now and hears whispered voices saying, 'Kill yourself.'"

Several months ago, the family had consulted with a psychiatrist who talked with the adolescent and prescribed an antipsychotic medication. It made her tired for several months, causing her to fail in school. Alarmed, the parents sought a second medical opinion.

The mother could not mask her worry. "Gabriela tells me she hears whispers when she goes to bed."

"It's a group of people who are whispering. I know it is coming from my mind," the daughter said. In other words, she was acknowledging that the whispers were self-condemning thoughts.

I was relieved. If Gabriela were hearing the "whispers" outside of herself, she might be experiencing a psychosis; however, her response informed me that she was obsessive, a less serious symptom and often associated with compulsions. Of further importance was that the "whispers" didn't occur in the daytime when she was occupied with tasks of daily living.

Gabriela's medical information listed a recent onset of stuttering, which was worse when she was anxious; yet, she didn't stutter during the interview, the EEG, or subsequent follow-ups.

Her physical exam, including a neurological screen, was within normal limits.

Asking patients "how they feel" doesn't provide a physician with objective information about their automatic brain function; however, examining their cognitive abilities can yield clues about their neurophysiology.

Gabriela could spell five-letter words forward and backward, a normal performance reflecting intact temporal lobes. Yet, she had difficulty repeating numbers in a sequence. In addition, her ability to recall a complex paragraph immediately was moderately impaired.

Having this information confirmed my next step. I discontinued the antipsychotic, and when the medication was eliminated from her body, I obtained a baseline EEG and QEEG. Her visual EEG was abnormally slow, and her quantitative EEG showed excessive voltages in lower alpha frequencies, a pattern that improves with up-regulation.

What Gabriela needed is a common amino acid, which is available in health food stores, quality supermarkets, and online.

Within a month of prescribing an amino acid, her sleep deprivation resolved, and the critical whispers, ordering her to kill herself, ceased. A follow-up EEG/QEEG appeared normal, and she soon returned to her prior level of functioning as an "A" student. After several additional months, another EEG/QEEG found even further improvement from the first post-treatment study. After nearly a year since her initial evaluation treatment, Gabriela is thriving.

This case is a blatant example of the risks and errors associated with assuming conclusions from a patient's symptoms, behaviors, and verbal descriptions of their mental distress. What is needed is information about individual brain function. This data can be a game changer.

CHAPTER 16

LESSONS LEARNED/CALL TO ACTION

Psychiatry is the only medical specialty that doesn't routinely measure the function of the organ that is the object of treatment, namely the brain. As a result, psychiatrists and other doctors who are guided only by the Diagnostic and Statistical Manual of Mental Disorders (DSM) are merely medicating symptoms and behaviors – without neurophysiologic measures – and have no objective way to learn from their mistakes and improve treatment.

Monitoring of automatic physical functions should be conducted:

1. Vital signs - pulse rate and blood pressure after sitting for 10 minutes. Refer to the standards set by the American College of Cardiology or the American Heart Association. Those parameters can be found on the Internet.
2. Sleep/wake cycle
3. Bowel transit time
4. Cognitive functions - simple math without paper

5. Diet – maintaining a healthy weight and balanced diet
6. Physical fitness – moderate exercise 3 to 4 times a week of 20 to 30 minutes
7. Medication – Prescribed medication by a physician should not cause adverse effects. A negative response to a prescribed medication should prompt a call to your doctor.

A person should be on the alert for any weight gain, difficulty in thinking, or sexual dysfunction. These are clues that one is not optimally medicated and further action is needed.

Medical research has taught me that some people are born with inherited differences in their automatic brain circuits. Despite advances in neuroscience and the fact that the decade of the brain was 30 years ago, psychiatry continues to ignore these individual brain differences/neuro-physiology in brain activity that cause physical and mental disorders. As a result, these conditions are often untreated or mistreated and cause unspeakable misery.

Since its inception, psychiatry has violated the medical model by labeling patients with troublesome repetitive symptoms and/or behaviors as mentally ill without conducting a comprehensive physical exam and monitoring their automatic nervous system. It is time to integrate the automatic physical functions along with EEG/QEEG measures across all medical specialties in the selection of effective treatment for each patient which is essential in improving physical health and mental wellbeing.

CHAPTER 17

I KNEW THERE WAS A BETTER WAY

Born a lefty, my first-grade teacher repeatedly beat my left hand and arm, as in the State of Virginia circa 1947, left handedness was considered sinister. The residual shame of being bullied and scorned probably influenced me in subtle ways into adulthood.

Being captain of the safety patrol in grade school temporarily elevated my social status, but my classmates did not overlook that I was chubby. It wasn't until my junior year of high school that I decreased my weight by 30 pounds. Then, the high school clubs invited me to join.

I did not.

When I became a licensed physician, I followed the medical model and physically examined patients during military service. Additionally, I had lab tests to guide me in the diagnosis and treatment of physical illnesses. I wondered about the invisible illnesses that plagued so many people. Could I help those with depression or anxiety? Were these symptoms strictly mental or generated by physical conditions? That question I would be able to answer years later.

When I became a psychiatrist, I abandoned the use of physical exams because psychiatrists were not taught to physically examine patients. Listening was – and still is - the focus. The Hippocratic Oath pledges to "Do No Harm," yet I was limited in the treatment options I had at my disposal. It was guessing when I prescribed medication. I knew I could do better.

A decade later, I learned about Dr. E. Roy John's research. His EEG/QEEG technology provided a new lab test that I could use to record each patient's brain activity. The information was objective data.

For the last 30 years I have not followed the psychiatric model. I did find a better, objective way and improved it over time. Treatment is based on individual physical findings and EEG/QEEG data. I am waiting for the psychiatric profession to catch up with my method. It works, just ask my patients.

For more information on how this can be achieved, the Brain1st™ method, and Dr. Hamlin Emory, visit www.dremory.com and www.emoryinstitute.org.

BIBLIOGRAPHY

Fall, Bernard B.; "Street Without Joy, The French Debacle in Indochina";
Originally published: Harrisburg, PA: Stackpole Co. 1961;
© 1961, 1963, 1964 by Bernard B. Fall; renewed in 1989
by Dorothy Fall; Stackpole Books, 5067 Ritter Road,
Mechanicsburg, PA 17055; wwwstackpolebooks.com; pg. 3-31

Diagnostic and Statistical Manual of Mental Disorders (DSM); editions
I – V; American Psychiatric Association

Freud, Sigmund; "Five Lectures on Psycho-Analysis, The Standard
Edition"; translated, edited and copyright © 1961 by James
Strachey; biographical introduction copyright © 1989 by Peter
Gay; W. Norton & Company, Inc.; 500 Fifth Avenue, New
York/London; pg. 3-62.

Ross, W.D. editor, revised by J.O. Urmson; Nicomachean Ethics, Books I –
X in Jonathan Barnes, editor; The Complete Works of Aristotle,
Volume Two; pg. 1729 – 1867; Bollingen Series LXXI; copyright
© 1984 by *The Jowett Copyright Trustees*; Princeton University
Press, 41 William St.; Princeton, New Jersey.

Cannon, Walter B.; The Wisdom of the Body; copyrights © 1932,
1960; revised, enlarged edition copyright © 1939 by Walter
B. Cannon; copyright renewed by Cornelia Cannon 1966,
1967; Preface xiii – xv; 324 pg.; Epilogue pg. 305 – 324; W.W.
Norton & Company, Inc.

Bacon, Francis; The New Organon; Author's Preface: pg. 2-4; Aphorisms;
pg. 6-20; Middletown, Delaware, USA; 2018.

John, ER, Karmel BZ, Corning WC, et al. Neurometrics. Science 196: 1393-1410; 1977.

Micale, Mark S., Editor; "Beyond the Unconscious, Essays of Henri F. Ellenberger in the History of Psychiatry"; Chapter 12, "The Fallacies of Psychiatric Classification", pg. 309 – 327; copyright © 1993 by Princeton University Press; Published by Princeton University Press, 41 Williams Street, Princeton, New Jersey 08540.

Niedermeyer, E. and Lopes Da Silva, F.; Electroencephalography, Fifth Edition; © 2005 by Lippincott Williams & Wilkins; 530 Walnut Street, Philadelphia, PA 19106 USA; LWW.com.

Engel, L. George; Romano, John; Ferris, Eugene B.; "Variations in the Normal Electroencephalogram during a Five-Year Period"; Science, New Series, Vol. 105, No. 2736; pg. 600-601; Jun 6, 1947.

Trzepacz, Paula T., Baker, Robert W., "The Psychiatric Mental Status Examination;" Oxford University Press, Inc.; 198 Madison Avenue, New York, New York 10016-4314; 196 pages; copyright ©1993.

Bos, Gerrit; "On Asthma", Volume I; "The Complete Medical Works of Moses Maimonides"; pgs. 84 & 91; Copyright ©2002 by Brigham Young University Press; Provo, Utah.

Eysenck, Hans J.; "The Biology of Personality"; New Preface by Sybil B.G. Eysenck; Transaction Publishers, Rutgers-The State University, 35 Berrue Circle, Piscataway, New Jersey 08854-8042. Chapter 2, The Structure of Personality; pg. 34-74.

Electroencephalography, Fifth Edition; Basic Principles, Clinical Applications, and Related Fields; Edited by Niedermeyer, Ernst and Lopes Da Silva, Fernando; Copyright © 2005 by Lippincott Williams & Wilkins; 530 Walnut Street, Philadelphia, PA 19106 USA.

Suffin, SC.; Emory, WH; "Neurometric Subgroups in Attentional and Affective Disorders and Their Association with Pharmacotherapeutic Outcome"; Clinical Electroencephalography; Vol. 26, No 2, pg. 76-83, 1995.

*[Nuwer, M. et al; American Academy of Neurology Position Paper on QEEG; 1997 or 1998] to be confirmed or negated asap

Martin, JB; "The Integration of Neurology, Psychiatry, and Neuroscience in the 21st Century"; Am J Psychiatry 159:695-704; May 2002.

Hughes, JR; Fino, John J; "EEG in Seizure Prognosis: Association of Slow Wave Activity and Other Factors in Patients with Apparent Misleading Epileptiform Findings"; Clinical EEG and
Neuroscience; Vol. 35, No. 4, pg. 181-184, 2004.

Suffin, SC; Emory, WH; Schiller, MJ; and Kling, A; "QEEG Database Method for Predicting Pharmacotherapeutic Outcome in Refractory Major Depression"; Journal of American Physicians and Surgeons. 2007; 12(4).

Groopman, J; "How Doctors Think"; Houghton Mifflin Company, Boston & New York; pg. 21 & 55; learning from medical errors; 2007.

Raichle, ME; "The Restless Brain"; Brain Connectivity; Vol. 1, Number 1, 2011; © Mary Ann Liebert, Inc.; DOI: 10.1089/brain.2011.0019.

Snyder, AZ and Raichle, ME; A Brief History of the Resting State: the Washington University Perspective; Neuroimage; August 15; 62(2): pg. 202-910; 2012.

Salinsky, MC; Oken, BS; Morehead, L; "Intraindividual analysis of antiepileptic drug effects on EEG background rhythms; Electroencephalography and Clinical Neurophysiology, 90 (1994); pg. 186-193; © 1994 Elsevier Science Ireland Ltd.

Emory, H; Wells, C; Mizrahi, N; "Quantitative EEG and Current Source Density Analysis of Combined Antiepileptic Drugs and Dopaminergic Agents in Genetic Epilepsy: Two Case Studies." Clinical EEG and Neuroscience. 2014; 1-7; published online Oct. 17.

Hampton, LM; Daubresse, M; Chang, HY; Alexander, GC; Budnitz, DS; "Emergency department visits by adults for psychiatric medication adverse events"; JAMA Psychiatry; Sept 71(9):1006-14; 2014.

Raichle, ME; "The restless brain: how intrinsic activity organizes brain function", Philosophical Transactions of the Royal Society B"; pg. 1-11, March 30, 2015.

Latvala, A., et al; "Association of Resting Heart Rate and Blood Pressure in Late Adolescence with Subsequent Mental Disorders"; JAMA Psychiatry. 2016; 73(12); pg. 1268-1275.

Kontopoulou, T.; Marketos, S.; "The Ancient Greek Origin of a Modern Scientific Principle"; Hormones 2002: 1(2):124-125.

Latvala, A.; Kuja-Halkola, R.; Almqvist, C.; Larsson, H.; Lichtenstein, P.; "A Longitudinal Study of Resting Heart Rate and Violent Criminality in More Than 7000,000 Men; JAMA Psychiatry 72(10); pg 971-978; 2015.

Emory, H., Wells, C. and Mizrahi, N.; Quantitative EEG and Current Source Density Analysis of Combined Antiepileptic Drugs and Dopamine Agents in Genetic Epilepsy: Two Case Studies; © EEG and Clinical Neuroscience Society; Clinical EEG and Neuroscience 1-7; 2014.

Emory, H. and Mizrahi, N.; Monoamine Oxidase Inhibition in a Patient with Type I Diabetes and Depression. Journal of Diabetes Science and Technology; pg. 1-2; sagepub.com/published online April 2016.

Emory H and Mizrahi N.; Glycaemic Control by Monoamine Oxidase Inhibition in a Patient with Type I Diabetes; Diabetes and Vascular Disease Research; pg. 1-3; © the authors; sagepub. co.uk/published online 2016.

Projections of National Expenditures for Treatment of Mental and Substance Use Disorders, 2010-2020; U.S. Department of Health and Human Services; Substance Abuse and Mental Health Services Administration (SAMHSA); www.samhsa.gov.

ACKNOWLEGEMENTS

Steve Suffin MD

Carl Cadwell DDS & Lynda

Meyer Proler MD

Mark Shatsky DO

John Whitworth

Bob Johnson

Lawanda Katzman Staenberg Ph.D.

Dick Van Dyke

E. Roy John Ph.D./Neurometrics

Cynthia H Rose (Morris), LMFT, LADC, CCTP - Book Title

Emory Institute Staff

Randy Bruner – Cover Design

Patients/Research

CURRICULUM VITAE
W. HAMLIN EMORY MD

Education
B.S. Washington and Lee University, 1959-1963
Lexington, Virginia

M.D. University of Virginia School of Medicine 1963-1967
Charlottesville, Virginia

Post-Graduate Training
Internship
Vanderbilt University Medical Center and Hospital 1967-1968
Nashville, Tennessee

Residency
Adult Psychiatry; VA Hospital 1972-1974
Brentwood, California

Fellowship
Child Psychiatry; Neuropsychiatric Institute 1974-1976
University of California, Los Angeles

Military Service
Flight Surgeon Trainee
Naval Aerospace Medical Institute 1968-1969
Pensacola, Florida
Naval Flight Surgeon
First Marine Air Group 1969-1970
Quang Tri, South Vietnam

Senior Medical Officer
U.S. Naval Air Facility; Sigonella, Sicily 1970-1972

Medical Director
Ventura Institute of Psychiatry 1977-2003
250 Lombard St.
Thousand Oaks, CA 91360

Ventura Institute of Psychiatry 1996-2007
436 North Bedford Drive
Beverly Hills, CA 90210

Emory Neurophysiologic Institute 2012-Present
2080 Century Park East; Suite 1409;
Los Angeles, CA 90067
www.emoryinstitute.org

Academic Appointment
Asst. Clinical Professor, Dept. of Psychiatry;
Geffen School of Medicine at UCLA 1976-Present

Licensures and Certifications (Active)
Certificate: American Board of Psychiatry and Neurology 1982

Medical License:State of California 1968

Memberships
American Medical Association 1993-Present
American Psychiatric Association 1993-Present
Clinical EEG and Neuroscience Society 1985-Present
SocietyforBrainMappingandTherapeutics 2016-Present

Publications:
1. Emory H, Mizrahi N. Glycaemic control by monoamine oxidase inhibition in a patient with type 1 diabetes; Diabetes and Vascular Disease Research 2017, Vol. 14(2) 163-165
2. Emory H, Mizrahi N. Monoamine Oxidase Inhibition in a Patient with Type I Diabetes & Depression; J Diabetes Sci

Technol. 1-2, Mar 8, 2016

3. Emory H, Wells C and Mizrahi N. Quantitative EEG and Current Source Density Analysis of Combined Antiepileptic Drugs and Dopaminergic Agents in Genetic Epilepsy: Two Case Studies. Clinical EEG and Neuroscience 1-7; published online Oct. 17, 2014.

4. Suffin SC, Emory WH, Schiller, MJ and Kling A. QEEG Database Method for Predicting Pharmacotherapeutic Outcome in Refractory Major Depressive Disorder. Journal of American Physicians and Surgeons. 2007; 12(4).

5. Suffin SC, Emory WH, Schiller, MJ and Kling A. QEEG Database Method for Predicting Pharmacotherapeutic Outcome in Refractory Major Depressive Disorder. J of American Physicians and Surgeons. 2007; 12(4).

6. Suffin, SC and Emory, WH. Neurometric Subgroups in Attentional and Affective Disorders and Their Associations with Pharmacotherapeutic Outcome. J of Clinical EEG 1995; 26:76-83.

7. Van Putten, T and Emory, WH. Traumatic Neurosis in Vietnam Returnees: A Forgotten Diagnosis? Archives of General Psychiatry. Nov. 1973; 29(5): 695-8.

Contributions:

1. Use of Referenced –EEG (rEEG) in assisting medication selection for the treatment of depression. DeBattista C, et.al., Journal of Psychiatric Research. 45 (2011) 64-75.

2. "The Eating Disorder Sourcebook" by Carolyn Costin M.A., M.Ed., M.F.T.

3. "The Military Setting" in Boredom, Roots of Discontent and Aggression. Editor: Goetzl, F. Grizzly Peak Press, 1975.

Professional Affiliations

Scientific Committee

Society for Brain Mapping & Therapeutics (SBMT) 2016-Present

Medical Director Emory Neurophysiologic Institute

2080 Century Park East; Suite 1409

Los Angeles, California 2012-Present

www.emoryinstitute.org

Asst. Clinical Professor Psychiatry
Geffen School of Medicine, UCLA, LA, CA 1976-Present

Board Member
CNS Response, Inc.; Santa Ana, CA 1999-2006

Licensures and Certifications (Active)
Certificate
American Board of Psychiatry and Neurology1982
Medical LicenseState of California 1968

Memberships
American Medical Association 1993-Present
American Psychiatric Association 1993-Present
Clinical EEG and Neuroscience Society 1985-Present

Lectures
1. Suffin SC and Emory WH. Neurometric EEG Classifiers and Response to Medicine. Symposium at the 1996 American Psychiatric Association Annual Meeting, Washington D.C.
2. Advancing Therapeutics of Brain-based Disorders; Medical Protocol and EEG Biomarkers Link Medical Treatment with Neurobiological Differences. Claremont Colleges Neuroscience Lecture Series, Oct. 20, 2006.
3. Finding and Fixing Brain Variations That Cause Physical Illnesses and Psychiatric Syndromes; Cadwell Laboratories; Tri-Cities WA; January 30, 2016
4. Inclusive Medical Approach with EEG & QEEG Features Predict Catecholamine Response in Idiopathic Genetic Epilepsies (IGE); SBMT Annual Meeting, Los Angeles Millennial Biltmore, April 18, 2017
5. Neuroplasticity in Medical Illnesses and Psychiatric Syndromes; SBMT Annual Meeting, Los Angeles Millennial Biltmore, April 20, 2017

Poster Presentations
1. Emory WH, Wells C and Mizrahi N. EEG Topography and LORETA Tomography in Neuropathology and Treatment of

Genetic Epilepsy. Proceedings: American Clinical Neurophysiology Society 2020 Annual Meeting; New Orleans, LA.

2.   Emory WH, Wells C and Mizrahi N. EEG Topography and LORETA Tomography in Neuropathology and Treatment of Genetic Epilepsy. Proceedings: 2013 Annual Meeting of the EEG and Clinical Neuroscience Society; University of Geneva; Switzerland.

3.   Emory WH, Shatsky ML, Wells CG. Questioning the Risk Profile of Selegiline Hydrochloride. Proceedings: 2012 Annual Meeting of the American Psychiatric Association.

4.   Emory WH, Shatsky ML, Wells CG. EEG and QEEG as Adjuncts to Clinical Assessment Predicts Response to Atypical Treatment Options. Proceedings: 2011 Annual Meeting of the American Neuropsychiatric Association.

5.   Suffin SC, Gutierrez NM, Karan S, Aurua G, Emory WH and Kling A. EEG Predicts Pharmacotherapeutic Outcome in Depressed Patients: A Prospective Trial. Program and Abstracts on New Research, Proceedings: 1997 Annual Meeting of the American Psychiatric Association; Washington D.C.

6.   Suffin SC, Emory WH and Proler ML. Neurometric Predictors of Response to Medication in Psychiatric Patients. Proceedings: 1997 American Clinical Neurophysiology Society; Bloomfield, CT.

Patents

1.   Suffin, Stephen C. (Sherman Oaks, CA, US), Emory, Hamlin W. (Malibu, CA, US), Brandt, Leonard (San Juan Capistrano, CA, US), (CNS Response) 2005. Compositions and methods for treatment of nervous system disorders. United States 20050118286. 2005-02-06.

2.   Suffin, Stephen C. (Sherman Oaks, CA, US), Emory, Hamlin W. (Malibu, CA, US), Brandt, Leonard (San Juan Capistrano, CA, US), (CNS Response) 2005. Compositions and methods for treatment of nervous system disorders. United States 20050096311. 2005-05-05.

3.   Suffin, Stephen C. (Sherman Oaks, CA, US), Emory, Hamlin W. (Malibu, CA, US), Brandt, Leonard J. (Laguna Hills, CA, US), (CNS Response, Inc.) 2009. Electroencephalography based systems and methods for selecting therapies and predicting outcomes. United States 7489964. 2009-10-02.

4. Suffin, Stephen C. (Sherman Oaks, CA, US), Emory, Hamlin W. (Malibu, CA, US), Brandt, Leonard J. (Laguna Hills, CA, US), (CNS Response, Inc.) 2008. Electroencephalography based systems and methods for selecting therapies and predicting outcomes. United States 20080125669. 2008-29-05.

5. Suffin, Stephen C. (Sherman Oaks, CA, US), Emory, Hamlin W. (Malibu, CA, US), Brandt, Leonard J. (San Juan Capistrano, CA, US), (CNS Response, Inc.) 2003. Electroencephalography based systems and methods for selecting therapies and predicting outcomes. United States 20030135128. 2003-17-07.

6. Suffin, Stephen C. (Sherman Oaks, CA, US), Emory, Hamlin W. (Malibu, CA, US), Brandt, Leonard J. (Laguna Hills, CA, US), (CNS Response, Inc.) 2007. Electroencephalography based systems and methods for selecting therapies and predicting outcomes. United States 7177675. 2007-13-02.

7. Suffin, Stephen C. (Sherman Oaks, CA, US), Emory, Hamlin W. (Malibu, CA, US), (CNS Response, Inc.) 2003. EEG prediction method for medication response. United States 20030144875. 2003-31-07.

8. Suffin, Stephen C. (Sherman Oaks, CA, US), Emory, Hamlin W. (Malibu, CA, US), (CNS Response, Inc.) 2005. EEG prediction method for medication response. United States 20050251419. 2005-10-02.

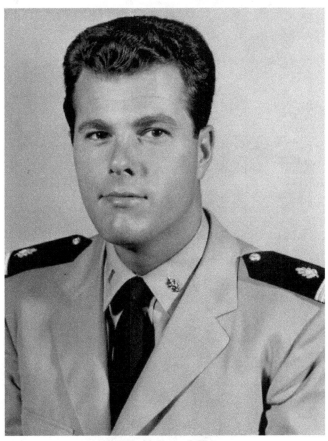

Hamlin Emory MD
Official U.S. Navy Photo
Late 1960's

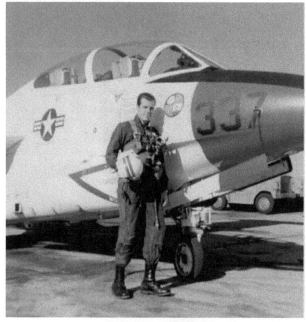

Hamlin Emory MD
Flight School 1969

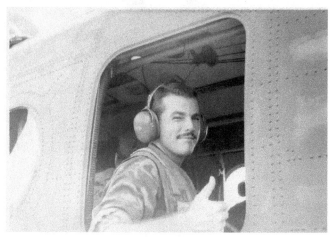

Hamlin Emory MD
Medevac Mission
Vietnam 1970

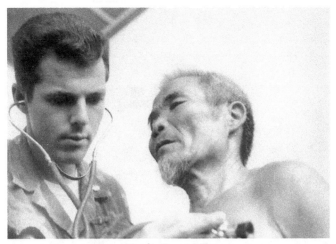

Hamlin Emory MD
Outpatient Clinic
Quang Tri, Vietnam 1970

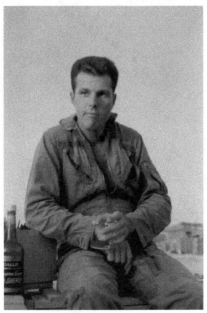

Hamlin Emory MD
"Taking a break"
Vietnam 1970

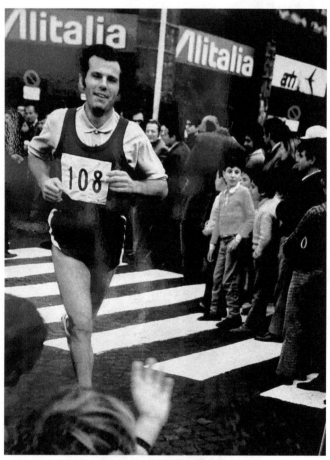

Hamlin Emory MD
10K Race in Catania, Italy 1970s

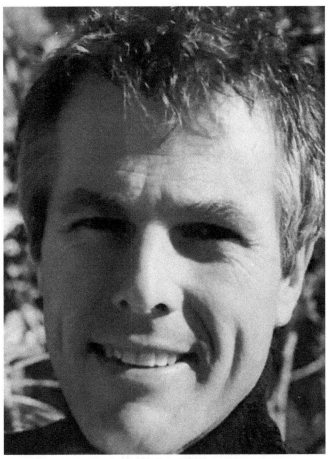

Hamlin Emory MD
Early 1990's

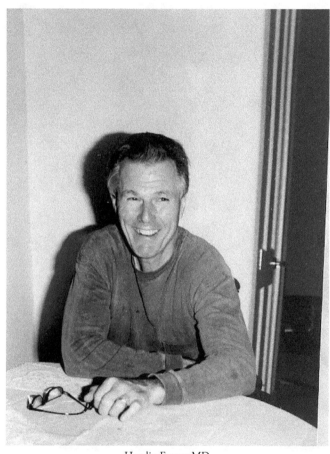

Hamlin Emory MD
Late 1990s

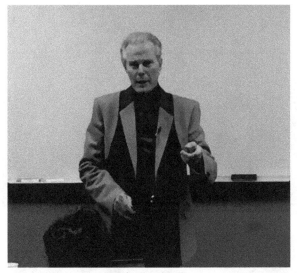

Hamlin Emory MD
Cadwell Laboratories Presentation 2016

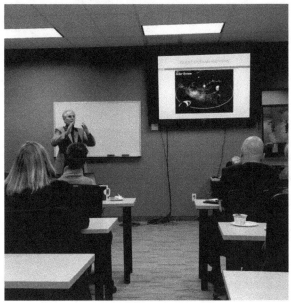

Hamlin Emory MD
Cadwell Laboratories Presentation 2016

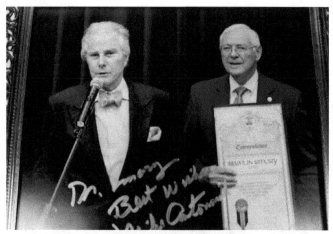

Hamlin Emory MD
Receives Commendation from City of Los Angeles 2016

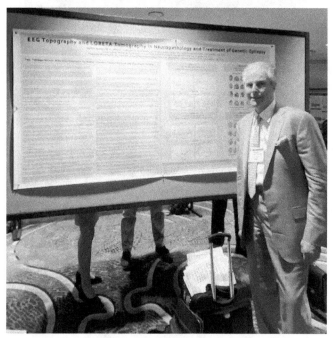

Hamlin Emory MD
Poster Presentation
New Orleans, 2020

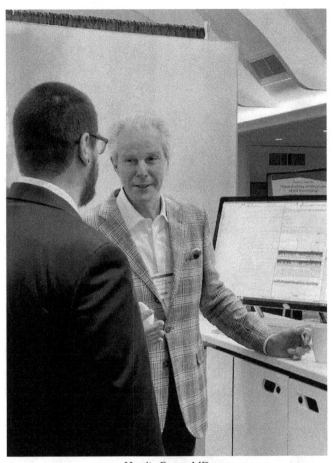

Hamlin Emory MD
Poster Presentation
New Orleans, 2020

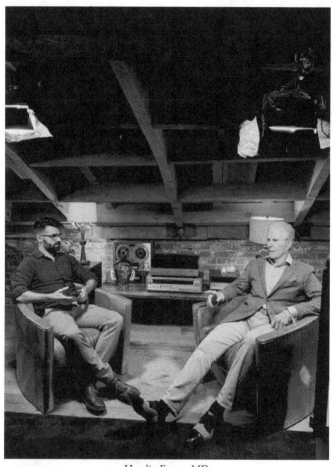

Hamlin Emory MD
Talk Show Appearance 2020